Cutaneous Malignancy

Editors

NICOLE R. LEBOEUF
CECILIA LAROCCA

HEMATOLOGY/ONCOLOGY CLINICS OF NORTH AMERICA

www.hemonc.theclinics.com

Consulting Editors
GEORGE P. CANELLOS
H. FRANKLIN BUNN

February 2019 • Volume 33 • Number 1

ELSEVIER

1600 John F. Kennedy Boulevard • Suite 1800 • Philadelphia, Pennsylvania, 19103-2899

http://www.theclinics.com

HEMATOLOGY/ONCOLOGY CLINICS OF NORTH AMERICA Volume 33, Number 1
February 2019 ISSN 0889-8588, ISBN 13: 978-0-323-65459-3

Editor: Stacy Eastman
Developmental Editor: Kristen Helm

Hematology/Oncology Clinics (ISSN 0889-8588) is published bimonthly by Elsevier Inc., 360 Park Avenue South, New York, NY 10010-1710. Months of issue are February, April, June, August, October, and December. Business and Editorial Offices: 1600 John F. Kennedy Blvd., Ste. 1800, Philadelphia, PA 19103–2899. Customer Service Office: 3251 Riverport Lane, Maryland Heights, MO 63043. Periodicals postage paid at New York, NY and at additional mailing offices. Subscription prices are $430.00 per year (domestic individuals), $830.00 per year (domestic institutions), $100.00 per year (domestic students/residents), $480.00 per year (Canadian individuals), $1028.00 per year (Canadian institutions) $547.00 per year (international individuals), $1028.00 per year (international institutions), and $255.00 per year (international and Canadian students/residents). International air speed delivery is included in all *Clinics* subscription prices. All prices are subject to change without notice. **POSTMASTER:** Send address changes to *Hematology/Oncology Clinics of North America*, Elsevier Health Sciences Division, Subscription Customer Service, 3251 Riverport Lane, Maryland Heights, MO 63043. Customer Service (orders, claims, online, change of address): Elsevier Health Sciences Division, Subscription **Customer Service, 3251 Riverport Lane, Maryland Heights, MO 63043. Tel: 1-800-654-2452 (U.S. and Canada); 314-447-8871 (outside U.S. and Canada). Fax: 314-447-8029. E-mail: journalscustomerservice-usa@elsevier.com (for print support); journalsonlinesupport-usa@elsevier.com (for online support).**

Reprints. For copies of 100 or more, of articles in this publication, please contact the Commercial Reprints Department, Elsevier Inc., 360 Park Avenue South, New York, New York 10010-1710; Tel.: 212-633-3874, Fax: 212-633-3820, E-mail: reprints@elsevier.com.

Hematology/Oncology Clinics of North America is covered in *MEDLINE/PubMed (Index Medicus), EMBASE/ Excerpta Medica, and BIOSIS.*

Contributors

CONSULTING EDITORS

GEORGE P. CANELLOS, MD
William Rosenberg Professor of Medicine, Department of Medical Oncology, Dana-Farber Cancer Institute, Boston, Massachusetts

H. FRANKLIN BUNN, MD
Professor of Medicine, Division of Hematology, Brigham and Women's Hospital, Harvard Medical School, Boston, Massachusetts

EDITORS

NICOLE R. LeBOEUF, MD, MPH
Assistant Professor, Department of Dermatology, Harvard Medical School, Clinical Director, The Centers for Melanoma and Cutaneous Oncology, Dana-Farber Cancer Institute, Dana-Farber/Brigham and Women's Cancer Center, Boston, Massachusetts

CECILIA LAROCCA, MD
Instructor, Department of Dermatology, Brigham and Women's Hospital, Dana-Farber Cancer Institute, Harvard Medical School, Boston, Massachusetts

AUTHORS

CHRISTINE S. AHN, MD
Department of Pathology, Wake Forest School of Medicine, Winston-Salem, North Carolina

OLEG E. AKILOV, MD, PhD
Director of Cutaneous Lymphoma Program, Assistant Professor, Department of Dermatology, University of Pittsburgh, Pittsburgh, Pennsylvania

MACKENZIE ASEL, MD
Department of Dermatology, The Centers for Melanoma and Cutaneous Oncology, Dana-Farber Cancer Institute, Boston, Massachusetts

MEHUL D. BHATT, MD, MBA
Department of Dermatology, University of Pennsylvania, Philadelphia, Pennsylvania

JOI B. CARTER, MD
Section of Dermatology, Dartmouth-Hitchcock Medical Center, Lebanon, New Hampshire

CYNTHIA CHEN, BS
Cutaneous Oncology Research Fellow, Columbia University Vagelos College of Physicians and Surgeons, New York, New York

FABIANA DAMASCO, MD
Fellow, Department of Dermatology, University of Pittsburgh, Pittsburgh, Pennsylvania

DAVID FISHER, MD
Assistant Professor of Medicine, Lymphoma Clinic, Dana-Farber Cancer Institute, Boston, Massachusetts

LARISA J. GESKIN, MD
Associate Professor, Department of Dermatology, Columbia University, New York, New York

AMRITA GOYAL, MD
Department of Dermatology, University of Minnesota, Minneapolis, Minnesota

YUHAN D. GU, BS
Cutaneous Oncology Research Fellow, Columbia University Vagelos College of Physicians and Surgeons, New York, New York

REBECCA I. HARTMAN, MD, MPH
Department of Dermatology, Brigham and Women's Hospital, Melanoma Program, Dana-Farber Cancer Institute, Boston, Massachusetts

ERIC D. JACOBSEN, MD
Clinical Director, Lymphoma Clinic, Dana-Farber Cancer Institute, Boston, Massachusetts

ALFRED BENNETT JENSON, MS, MD
James Graham Brown Cancer Center, University of Louisville School of Medicine, Louisville, Kentucky

JAE YEON JUNG, MD, PhD
Division of Dermatology, University of Louisville School of Medicine, Onco-Dermatology Program, Norton Cancer Institute, Louisville, Kentucky

NANCY KADDIS, MD, MPH
Department of Hematology and Oncology, Dana-Farber Cancer Institute at St Elizabeth's Medical Center, Brighton, Massachusetts

DENNIS P. KIM, MD
Fellow, Mohs Micrographic Surgery, Brigham and Women's Faulkner Hospital, Jamaica Plain, Massachusetts

THOMAS KUPPER, MD
Chair, Department of Dermatology, Brigham and Women's Hospital, Dana-Farber Cancer Institute, Thomas B. Fitzpatrick Professor, Harvard Medical School, Boston, Massachusetts

KYLEE J.B. KUS, BS
Oakland University William Beaumont School of Medicine, Rochester, Minnesota

CECILIA LAROCCA, MD
Instructor, Department of Dermatology, Brigham and Women's Hospital, Dana-Farber Cancer Institute, Harvard Medical School, Boston, Massachusetts

ROBERT E. LeBLANC, MD
Department of Pathology and Laboratory Medicine, Dartmouth-Hitchcock Medical Center, Lebanon, New Hampshire

NICOLE R. LᴇBOEUF, MD, MPH
Assistant Professor, Department of Dermatology, Harvard Medical School, Clinical Director, The Centers for Melanoma and Cutaneous Oncology, Dana-Farber Cancer Institute, Dana-Farber/Brigham and Women's Cancer Center, Boston, Massachusetts

JENNIFER Y. LIN, MD
Department of Dermatology, Brigham and Women's Hospital, Melanoma Program, Dana-Farber Cancer Institute, Boston, Massachusetts

VINOD E. NAMBUDIRI, MD, MBA
Department of Dermatology, Brigham and Women's Hospital, Cutaneous Oncology Program, Dana-Farber Cancer Institute, Boston, Massachusetts

EMILY RUIZ, MD, MPH
Director, High-Risk Skin Cancer Clinic, Dana-Farber/Brigham and Women's Cancer Center, Associate Physician, Mohs and Dermatologic Surgery Center, Brigham and Women's Faulkner Hospital, Instructor, Harvard Medical School, Jamaica Plain, Massachusetts

OMAR P. SANGÜEZA, MD
Professor, Department of Pathology, Wake Forest School of Medicine, Winston-Salem, North Carolina

CHRYSALYNE SCHMULTS, MD, MSCE
Department of Dermatology, Brigham and Women's Hospital, Associate Professor, Harvard Medical School, Boston, Massachusetts

JOHN D. STRICKLEY, BS
James Graham Brown Cancer Center, University of Louisville School of Medicine, Louisville, Kentucky; Department of Dermatology, Center for Cancer Immunology and Cutaneous Biology Research Center, MGH Cancer Center, Massachusetts General Hospital, Harvard Medical School, Boston, Massachusetts

MANISHA THAKURIA, MD
Department of Dermatology, Brigham and Women's Hospital, Instructor of Dermatology, Harvard Medical School, Co-Director, Merkel Cell Carcinoma Center of Excellence, The Center for Cutaneous Oncology, Dana-Farber/Brigham and Women's Cancer Center, Boston, Massachusetts

ABIGAIL WALDMAN, MD, MHS
Department of Dermatology, Brigham and Women's Hospital, Instructor, Harvard Medical School, Boston, Massachusetts

YUN XUE, MD
Department of Dermatology, Brigham and Women's Hospital, Harvard Medical School, Boston, Massachusetts

Contents

missed diagnosis due to the wide histopathologic differential diagnosis of malignant small blue cell tumors. The advent of immunohistochemistry staining for cytokeratin 20, a shared neuroendocrine marker, greatly improved diagnostic accuracy. Over the past decade, staging, treatment, and surveillance of the cancer have progressed at a remarkably rapid pace. Herein, the authors provide an update on the current guidelines around diagnosis and management and review the exciting advancements on the horizon.

Malignant sweat gland neoplasms are a confusing area within dermatopathology, with many entities reported under several designations in the literature. This review describes the key clinical and histopathologic features of select malignant adnexal neoplasms, including porocarcinoma, papillary carcinoma, adenoid cystic carcinoma, cribriform carcinoma, apocrine hidradenocarcinoma, malignant mixed tumor of the skin, syringoid carcinoma, cylindrocarcinoma, spiradenocarcinoma, mucinous carcinoma, polymorphous sweat gland carcinoma, microcystic adnexal carcinoma, secretory carcinoma of the skin, and primary cutaneous signet ring cell carcinoma. For entities with overlapping features, differential diagnoses are discussed.

Extramammary Paget disease (EMPD) is a rare cutaneous malignancy most commonly affecting the genitals, perineum, and perianal area of the elderly. Despite its rarity, to those impacted, the disease and its treatment can have a tremendous impact on quality of life. Commonly confined to the epidermis, EMPD can be invasive, associated with contiguous extension or upward pagetoid spread of underlying malignancy or with distant synchronous malignancy. Because of its association with other cancers, formal evaluation is warranted. Treatment varies widely and evidence-based approaches are lacking. The authors review the workup and management options for the patient with EMPD.

Cutaneous sarcomas are rare malignancies that may present with a variety of clinical manifestations. This article focuses on 4 of the most common cutaneous sarcomas (Kaposi sarcoma, cutaneous angiosarcoma, dermatofibrosarcoma protuberans, and cutaneous leiomyosarcoma) and reviews clinical, diagnostic, and therapeutic aspects of these rare skin malignancies.

Cutaneous T-cell lymphomas are a heterogeneous collection of non-Hodgkin lymphomas that arise from skin-tropic memory T lymphocytes.

Among them, mycosis fungoides (MF) and Sézary syndrome (SS) are the most common malignancies. Diagnosis requires the combination of clinical, pathologic, and molecular features. Significant advances have been made in understanding the genetic and epigenetic aberrations in SS and to some extent in MF. Several prognostic factors have been identified. The goal of treatment is to minimize morbidity and limit disease progression. However, hematopoietic stem cell transplantation, considered for patients with advanced stages, is the only therapy with curative intent.

Primary cutaneous CD30$^+$ lymphoproliferative diseases (LPDs) comprise a range of diseases (LyP, pcALCL, and borderline lesions) with broad histologic and phenotypical characteristics, although they all share the common feature of a favorable prognosis notwithstanding histology suggestive of a high-grade lymphoma. Given their cytomorphologic similarities, accurate diagnosis and workup are needed to differentiate these distinct entities in order to best use novel biologic therapies and avoid aggressive overtreatment. Moreover, although CD30$^+$ LPDs have a favorable prognosis, secondary malignancies should be considered as part of the initial evaluation, and patients should have ongoing surveillance.

Rare lymphoma includes the entities that occur in less than 1% of cases of all lymphomas. Although the percentage is low, there are more than eight lymphomas classified as rare lymphomas. This article describes clinical presentation, diagnosis, prognosis, and management of the most common rare lymphomas, including primary cutaneous γδ T-cell lymphoma, primary cutaneous CD4$^+$ small/medium T-cell lymphoproliferative disorder, primary cutaneous acral CD8$^+$ T-cell lymphoma, primary cutaneous CD8$^+$ aggressive epidermotropic cytotoxic T-cell lymphoma, extranodal NK-/T-cell lymphoma, nasal type, and subcutaneous panniculitis-like T-cell lymphoma.

Primary cutaneous B-cell lymphomas are non-Hodgkin lymphomas that present in the skin without evidence of extracutaneous involvement at diagnosis. There are 3 types of primary cutaneous B-cell lymphomas: primary cutaneous marginal zone lymphoma, primary cutaneous follicle center lymphoma, and primary cutaneous diffuse large B-cell lymphoma, leg-type. Because it is most frequently diagnosed on skin biopsy, intravascular large B-cell lymphoma is commonly included with pcBCL. A complicating factor in diagnosing primary cutaneous B-cell lymphomas is that they can appear histologically identical to their extracutaneous counterparts. This review summarizes the clinical presentation, histopathology, evaluation, treatment, and differential diagnosis of these lymphomas.

In reviewing cutaneous manifestations of various hematologic malignancies, the authors focus on secondary cutaneous lymphomas and cutaneous manifestations of histiocyte disorders. Secondary cutaneous lymphomas are defined as skin lesions that develop secondary to infiltration by systemic lymphomas with predominantly extracutaneous involvement. In their review of histiocytic disorders with skin involvement, the authors focus on Langerhans cell histiocytosis and Rosai-Dorfman disease. Their review emphasizes the histology, pathophysiology, clinical presentation, prognosis, and treatments available for these diseases.

Although rare, cutaneous metastases portend a poor prognosis and are often an indicator of widespread disease. Breast cancer and melanoma are the most common types of cancer that are associated with spread to and within the skin; however, other malignancies, such as lung, colon, head and neck, and hematologic, have been described with a degree of relative frequency. A variety of clinical appearances and syndromes of cutaneous metastases are presented and described in this article. Possible treatment options, including skin-directed therapies and immunotherapies, are also discussed.

HEMATOLOGY/ONCOLOGY CLINICS OF NORTH AMERICA

SERIES OF RELATED INTEREST

Surgical Oncology Clinics of North America

THE CLINICS ARE AVAILABLE ONLINE!
Access your subscription at:
www.theclinics.com

Erratum

For the article on "First-Generation and Second-Generation Bruton Tyrosine Kinase Inhibitors in Waldenström Macroglobulinemia" in the October 2018 issue of *Hematology/Oncology Clinics of North America* (Volume 32, Issue 5), Dr. M. Lia Palomba's last name was erroneously excluded.

The online version of this issue has been corrected.

Hematol Oncol Clin N Am 33 (2019) xiii
https://doi.org/10.1016/j.hoc.2018.11.001
0889-8588/18/© 2018 Elsevier Inc. All rights reserved.

Preface

Cutaneous Malignancy

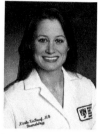
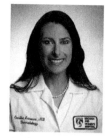

Nicole R. LeBoeuf, MD, MPH   Cecilia Larocca, MD
Editors

The skin is responsible for protecting us from temperature extremes, ultraviolet radiation, physical injury, and infection. As such, it is a complex and rich organ composed of diverse cell types, which have differentiated from the ectoderm, mesoderm, and neural crest. Malignancies that arise in the skin may originate from keratinocytes, melanocytes, Merkel cells, endothelial cells, adnexal structures, constituents of the connective tissue stroma, and skin-resident immune cells among others. The skin is also a common site for metastasis. Cutaneous malignancies range from indolent to among the most aggressive cancers encountered in oncology. They often require a multidisciplinary approach for treatment. The successful treatment of melanoma with immunotherapy has established the discipline of immune-oncology, which has led to a treatment renaissance across all solid and hematologic malignancies. With an understanding of the diverse normal and malignant cell types that may present in the most accessible site in the body, we are provided with a profound opportunity to investigate novel topical and intralesional immunotherapies, which, given the skin's rich immune milieu, may have synergistic effects when combined with immune checkpoint inhibitors, and targeted and conventional therapies. In this issue, the reader will review the clinical presentation, evaluation and management of the vast array of malignancies that present in the skin.

Nicole R. LeBoeuf, MD, MPH
Harvard Medical School
Department of Dermatology
Center for Cutaneous Oncology
Dana-Farber/Brigham and Women's Cancer Center
450 Brookline Avenue
Boston, MA 02115, USA

Hematol Oncol Clin N Am 33 (2019) xv–xvi
https://doi.org/10.1016/j.hoc.2018.09.007
0889-8588/19/© 2018 Published by Elsevier Inc.

hemonc.theclinics.com

Cecilia Larocca, MD
Harvard Medical School
Department of Dermatology
Center for Cutaneous Oncology
Dana-Farber/Brigham and Women's Cancer Center
450 Brookline Avenue
Boston, MA 02115, USA

E-mail addresses:
nleboeuf@bwh.harvard.edu (N.R. LeBoeuf)
clarocca@bwh.harvard.edu (C. Larocca)

Cutaneous Squamous Cell Carcinoma

Abigail Waldman, MD, MHS*, Chrysalyne Schmults, MD, MSCE

KEYWORDS

- Cutaneous squamous cell carcinoma • Treatment • Diagnosis • Skin cancer

KEY POINTS

- Cutaneous squamous cell carcinoma (cSCC) is a common skin cancer that presents as a scaly, red, or bleeding lesion on sun-exposed areas.
- UV exposure, fair skin, and immunosuppression increase incidence of cSCC.
- Recurrence and metastasis are associated with tumor diameter greater than 2 cm, depth greater than 2 mm or beyond subcutaneous fat, extensive or large-caliber perineural involvement, and poor differentiation on histopathology.
- AJCC 8 is used for TNM staging for cSCC of the head and neck. BWH offers an alternative T staging system.
- Management is primarily surgical with rare indications for adjuvant chemoradiation based on risk factors.

INCIDENCE AND EPIDEMIOLOGY

Cutaneous squamous cell carcinoma (cSCC) is the second most common nonmelanoma skin cancer. It accounts for 20% of skin cancer and results in 1 million cases in the United States each year resulting in up to 9000 estimated deaths.[1–4]

Depending on the latitude, the incidence of cSCC ranges from 5 to 499 per 100,000 patients.[5–8] The lifetime risk of developing SCC is 14–20% in a non-hispanic white population in the United States.[9,10] This number continues to increase annually with an estimated 50% to 200% increase in incidence in the last three decades and will likely continue to increase because of the aging population.[11]

CLINICAL PRESENTATION

cSCC presents as a red scaly plaque, typically in sun-exposed areas. Lesions are typically solitary (**Fig. 1**A); however, they rarely can present as multiple "in transit" metastases (**Fig. 1**B).

Disclosure Statement: No disclosures.
Department of Dermatology, Brigham and Women's Hospital, 1153 Centre Street, Suite 4J, Boston, MA 02130, USA
* Corresponding author.
E-mail address: awaldman10@bwh.harvard.edu

Hematol Oncol Clin N Am 33 (2019) 1–12
https://doi.org/10.1016/j.hoc.2018.08.001
0889-8588/19/

hemonc.theclinics.com

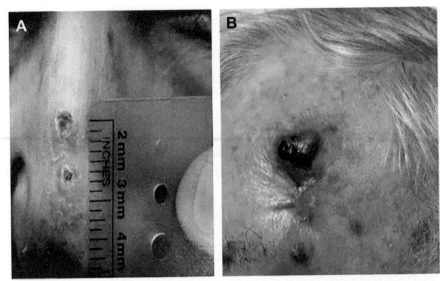

Fig. 1. Clinical presentation of SCC. (*A*) Primary locally invasive cSCC. (*B*) Multiple nodules representing in transit metastases.

WORK-UP

Diagnosis is made by a skin biopsy deep enough to allow the pathologist to comment on depth of invasion, perineural or lymphovascular invasion, differentiation, and connection to the overlying epidermis.[12] Local lymph nodes and parotid when appropriate should be evaluated by clinical examination and should be sampled if clinically involved.[13] The value of sentinel lymph node biopsy in cSCC without clinically apparent lymph nodes is currently unknown.[14–17] The patient should also be assessed for nerve involvement signified by neurologic pain or palsy. Generally, imaging is not required unless the clinical picture is suggestive of involvement of large-caliber nerves, muscle or bone, lymph node involvement, or when high-risk features are present.[12,13] When indicated, compute tomography with contrast is useful for evaluation of lymph node, soft tissue, or bone involvement. MRI is preferred to evaluate perineural invasion or orbital and intracranial extension.[18]

HISTOPATHOLOGY

On histopathology, cSCC differentiation may vary from well to poorly differentiated. Well-differentiated tumors exhibit interconnecting follicular infundibular type squamous epithelium. Mitosis may be rare or absent. Poor differentiation indicates that it is difficult to determine a keratinocyte lineage (**Fig. 2**).[19,20]

Low- or Moderate-Risk Histologic Variants

- Keratoacanthomas: a well-differentiated squamous proliferation with a crateriform appearance
- Verrucous carcinomas: well-differentiated SCC with prominent hyperkeratosis and "club-like tongues" of intradermal growth
- Clear cell: greater than 25% squamoid epithelial cells with cytoplasmic vacuolation (PAS+[periodic acid-schiff])

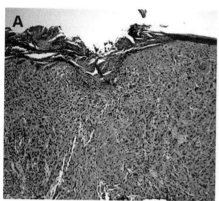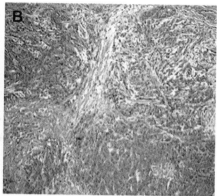

Fig. 2. Histopathology of cSCC. (*A*) (hematoxylin-eosin, original magnification ×4). (*B*) (hematoxylin-eosin, original magnification ×10).

Higher Risk Histologic Variants

- Acantholytic SCC: well-differentiated SCC with acantholysis
- Spindle cell SCC is a poorly differentiated variant with closely packed fascicles of pleomorphic spindle cells with high mitotic activity
- Adenosquamous carcinoma: mixed squamous and glandular differentiation originating from epidermis with interconnecting nests of anaplastic squamoid cells and desmoplastic stroma with 5% to 80% glandular differentiation (highlighted with CEA and CK7 immunostaining)

Uncommon Variants

- SCC with sarcomatoid differentiation
- Lymphoepithelioma-like carcinoma
- Pseudovascular SCC
- SCC with osteoclast-like giant cells

Immunohistochemistry is not typically needed except in the cases of poorly differentiated SCC or uncommon variants. Cutaneous SCC stains positive with p63, p40, MUC1 (epithelial membrane antigen), CK5/6, MNF116, and high-molecular weight 34 E12. BerEp4 should be negative in SCC.[20]

RISK FACTORS

The most significant risk factors resulting in cSCC include UV exposure, older age, fair skin (Fitzpatrick skin types I-III), and immunosuppression. UV (primarily UV-B) from the sun or tanning beds induces skin cancer by causing DNA damage.[21-25] The incidence of SCC doubles with each 8° to 10° in latitude.[26,27] Skin types that burn after UV exposure (related to Fitzpatrick skin type) are predisposed to developing cSCC.[28]

Other Risk Factors

cSCC is more common in men than women (3:1 ratio). The incidence increases with age, with an average age of onset in the mid-60s.[29] Immunosuppression can play a major role in cSCC, with solid transplant recipients suffering 65 to 250 times the risk of cSCC compared with the general population.[30-33] The rate of cSCC formation is related to the number of immunosuppressive agents, the type of immunosuppressant agent, and the amount of sun exposure or skin cancers before transplant.[32] Patients with chronic lymphocytic leukemia have an 8- to 10-fold increased risk for developing cSCC.[34,35] Patients exposed to vismodegib have eight times the risk of cSCC compared with control patients.[36]

Rare Risk Factors

Oncogenic human papillomavirus types 16 and 18 are associated with periungual and anogenital cSCC.[37] Environmental exposures associated with cSCC include arsenic, polycyclic aromatic hydrocarbons (tar, pitch, and soot), nitrosamines, and alkylating agents. Any exposure to ionizing radiation is associated with more aggressive cSCC, with high rates of recurrence and a 10% to 30% rate of metastasis.[38,39] The presence of rare familial syndromes (including xeroderma pigmentosum, albinism, epidermolysis bullosa, epidermolysis verruciformis, Ferguson Smith epithelioma, Rothmund-Thomson syndrome, Bloom syndrome) can predispose an individual to multiple cSCCs at a young age.[40]

GENETICS

cSCC carries more mutations than other common malignancies, with more than four times the mutation rates in melanoma.[41] Tumor protein 53 (TP53),[42] cyclin-dependent kinase inhibitor 2A mutations (CDKN2A), Ras mutations, and mutations of Notch homolog 1 are involved in cSCC carcinogenesis.[41,43] Genetic mutations found to be differentially expressed in cSCC include CXCL8 (IL8), MMP1, HIF1A, ITGA6, and ITGA2.[20,44]

MORTALITY

Although most cSCC are treated locally with no sequelae, a small subset result in tumor-specific mortality. In the United States, the annual disease-specific mortality is estimated to be 1.5% to 2% with up to 4% mortality rates reported in other countries; 5604 to 12,572 people with cSCC developed nodal metastases with an estimated 9000 deaths.[2,45] Factors associated with local recurrence and metastases are listed in **Table 1**.

Diameter

A tumor diameter greater than 2.0 cm doubles the risk of cSCC recurrence and triples the rate of metastasis compared with lesions less than 2 cm in diameter. Tumor

Table 1
cSCC tumor characteristics that increase the risk of recurrence and/or metastasis

Risk Factors	Recurrence	Metastasis
Diameter >2 cm	2 times	3 times
Depth >2 mm or beyond subcutaneous fat	10 times	11 times
Perineural involvement (>0.1 mm caliber nerve)	23 times	12 times
Poor differentiation	3 times	2 times
Recurrent	2–3 times	Up to 23 times for certain sites (ear/lip)
Site	2 times (ear)	3 times (ear), 5 times (vermillion/mucosal lip)
Arising in scar	not available	12 times
Immunosuppression	6 times	2 times

diameter greater than 2 cm is the risk factor most highly associated with disease-specific death and a 19-fold higher risk of death from cSCC compared with tumors less than 2 cm.[46]

Depth

Depth of disease is highly associated with recurrence and metastasis, with tumors of Breslow thickness greater than 2 mm having a 10-fold higher risk of local recurrence and tumors extending beyond subcutaneous fat having a local recurrence rate of 28% and an 11-fold higher risk of metastasis compared with more superficial tumors.[4,46,47]

Perineural Involvement

The overall incidence of perineural involvement in cSCC is 2% to 14%.[48,49] Perineural invasion of large-caliber nerves (involved nerves measuring ≥0.1 mm) is associated with increased nodal metastases and disease-specific mortality.[49,50] Tumors with large-caliber perineural invasion have local recurrence and metastatic risks of 47% and 35%, respectively, after wide local excision.[48,51]

Differentiation

The presence of poor differentiation indicates a poorer prognosis, with local recurrence risk more than triple when compared with well differentiation (7% vs 2%) and a metastatic risk approximately double (7% vs 3%) that of well-differentiated cSCCs.[4]

Previously Treated/Recurrent Cutaneous Squamous Cell Carcinoma

Once a cSCC has recurred, it has a much worse prognosis, with risk of spread to regional lymph nodes and distant metastases cited as 45% for ear cSCC and 32% for lip SCC.[51] Recurrent cSCCs are two to three times as likely to recur again after excisional surgery and Mohs micrographic surgery when compared with primary tumors.[52]

Site

cSCC of the ear has been reported to have a local recurrence risk of 5% after Mohs micrographic surgery, 19% after non-Mohs modalities, and a metastatic risk of 9% after greater than 5 years of follow-up. SCC of the lip has a reported metastatic risk of 14% after greater than 5 years of follow-up.[51,53]

Cutaneous Squamous Cell Carcinoma Arising in Scar

cSCCs arising from a leg ulcer, burn scar, radiation dermatitis, and other chronic wounds have a reported metastatic risk of 26%.[51]

Immunosuppression

cSCCs in immunosuppressed patients may display more rapid growth; recur locally in 13% of patients; and have a 5% to 8% risk of metastasis, usually in the second year after excision.[54–56] Prognosis is usually worse for older patients with tumors located on head and neck skin, when multiple tumors are present, and when there is a history of high exposure to the sun.[57–61]

STAGING
American Joint Committee on Cancer-8

In October 2016, the American Joint Committee on Cancer (AJCC) introduced the eighth edition of its cancer staging systems.[62] The AJCC-8 staging system classifies cSCC of the head and neck by local tumor burden (T), nodal status (N), and metastatic disease (M).[61,63] Stage T1 are tumors less than 2 cm. T2 are tumors 2–3.9 cm. T3 tumors are ≥4 cm or with minor bone erosion or large caliber perineural invasion or deep invasion >6 mm. T4a tumors invade to cortical bone or marrow and T4b invade the skull base or skull base foramen.

Brigham and Women's Hospital Tumor Classification System

The Brigham and Women's Hospital staging system, proposed in 2013, offers an alternative tumor (T) classification system but does not include N or M staging criteria.[64] High-risk features in this T classification system include tumor diameter greater than or equal to 2 cm, tumor invasion beyond the subcutaneous fat, perineural invasion of nerves greater than or equal to 0.1 mm in caliber, and poor differentiation. T stage is assigned as follows: T1, no high-risk features; T2a, one high-risk feature; T2b, two to three high-risk features; and T3, all four high-risk features or bone invasion.[62]

TREATMENT

cSCC is stratified into low risk or high risk. Guidelines are available to help guide treatment including those by the National Comprehensive Cancer Network (NCCN)[13] and the American Academy of Dermatology (AAD) guidelines (**Table 2**).[12]

There are two main types of margin analysis commonly used for surgically excised cSCC: sectional assessment used in standard excision, and complete circumferential peripheral and deep margin assessment (CCPDMA). Sectional assessment describes traditional "bread loaf" assessment and allows for visual assessment of approximately 1% of the marginal surface of a specimen, whereas CCPDMA involves en face sectioning that allows for histologic examination of nearly 100% of the marginal surface. The two main methods of CCPDMA used in keratinocyte carcinomas are Mohs micrographic surgery and the Tubingen method.

According to AAD and NCCN guidelines, for local low-risk SCC, first-line treatments include standard excision with 4- to 6-mm clinical margins and postoperative margin assessment.[12,13] For standard excision, recurrence rates are 8.10% for primary low-risk SCC.[51] If margins are positive, additional re-excision or Mohs surgery is considered depending on the location[13] For small tumors not in hair-bearing areas, curettage and electrodessication may be indicated.[12,65,66] Unlike in situ disease, no data support the use of cryotherapy, topical creams, or photodynamic therapy for the primary treatment of dermally invasive SCC.[12]

For high-risk cSCC, the AAD and NCCN guidelines recommend Mohs micrographic surgery, which boasts a 3% recurrence rate for primary cSCC and significantly improved outcomes for high-risk SCCs compared with standard assessment (see **Table 2**).[12,13,51]

Table 2
Mohs micrographic surgery versus standard "bread loaf" pathology assessment recurrence rates

	Mohs, %	Standard Excision, %
Primary cSCC	3.10	8.10
Recurrent SCC	10	23
Perineural involvement	0	47
SCC >2 cm	25.20	41.70
Poorly differentiated	32.60	53.60

Data from Rowe DE, Carroll RJ, Day CL Jr. Prognostic factors for local recurrence, metastasis, and survival rates in squamous cell carcinoma of the skin, ear, and lip. Implications for treatment modality selection. J Am Acad Dermatol 1992;26(6):976–90.

NCCN guidelines state that other measures of CCPDMA, such as the Tubingen method, can be used. When CCPDMA is not available, wide local excision with delayed closure is acceptable. Radiation should only be used as primary treatment in those patients who are not surgical candidates.[13] Radiation may be used as adjuvant therapy in some cases where extensive perineural invasion or large-caliber nerve invasion is present. Multidisciplinary approach is taken when positive margins are noted after Mohs micrographic surgery.[12,13]

Management for local regional or distant metastatic cSCC requires multidisciplinary involvement. NCCN recommends excision ± lymphadenectomy or parotidectomy when lymph nodes are involved.[13,67] Adjuvant chemoradiation may be considered pending margin evaluation or if extracapsular extension of lymph nodes is noted.[13,17,68,69] The AAD offers specific recommendations of epidermal growth factor receptor inhibitors or cisplatin when systemic therapy is needed; however, therapy is constantly evolving. The NCCN recommends consideration of clinical trials and anti-PD1 immunotherapy (eg. pembrolizumab, cemiplimab) is under active investigation.[12,70–74] For inoperable disease, chemoradiation plus palliative care is recommended. However, a recent study showed no benefit for chemoradiation with carboplatin based chemotherapy over radiation alone.[11,69]

PREVENTION

Photoprotective measures including sunscreen application have been shown to decrease SCC by 40%.[75,76] Other measures of prevention include those aimed at managing field cancerization (large defects of DNA damaged skin): 5-fluorouracil, imiquimod, topical retinoids, diclofenac sodium, ingenol mebutate, chemotherapy wraps, photodynamic therapy, nicotinamide and acitretin or capecitabine for very high-risk, immunosuppressed patients.[12]

MONITORING

A patient with at least one cSCC is at risk for additional cSCC and other for skin cancers, including basal cell carcinoma and melanoma.[77,78] The 5-year probability of another non-melanoma skin cancer (NMSC) after diagnosis of a first is 40.7%, the 10 year is 59.6%, and after more than one cSCC it is 82% and 91.2%.[79] After a diagnosis of local SCC, the NCCN guidelines suggest follow-up and screening every 3 to 12 months for 2 years after initial diagnosis and then every 2 years. For regional disease, suggested follow-up is every 1 to 3 months for 1 year, every 2 to 4 months for second year, every 4 to 6 months for the third year, and then every 6 to 12 months for life.[13,80] Concurrent patient and family member self-surveillance for cSCC and other skin cancers may be of additional utility in detecting new primary tumors.[81]

REFERENCES

1. Rogers HW, Weinstock MA, Feldman SR, et al. Incidence estimate of nonmelanoma skin cancer (keratinocyte carcinomas) in the U.S. population, 2012. JAMA Dermatol 2015;151(10):1081–6.
2. Karia P. Cutaneous squamous cell carcinoma: estimated incidence of disease, nodal metastasis, and deaths from disease in the United States, 2012. J Am Acad Dermatol 2013;68:957–66.
3. Schmults C. Factors predictive of recurrence and death from cutaneous squamous cell carcinoma. A 10-year, single-institution cohort study. JAMA Dermatol 2013;149:541–7.

4. Brantsch K. Analysis of risk factors determining prognosis of cutaneous squamous cell carcinoma: a prospective study. Lancet Oncol 2008;9:713–20.

5. Brewster DH, Bhatti LA, Inglis JH, et al. Recent trends in incidence of nonmelanoma skin cancers in the east of Scotland, 1992-2003. Br J Dermatol 2007; 156(6):1295–300.

6. Andersson EM, Paoli J, Wastensson G. Incidence of cutaneous squamous cell carcinoma in coastal and inland areas of Western Sweden. Cancer Epidemiol 2011;35(6):e69–74.

7. Staples MP, Elwood M, Burton RC, et al. Non-melanoma skin cancer in Australia: the 2002 national survey and trends since 1985. Med J Aust 2006;184(1):6–10.

8. Nguyen KD, Han J, Li T, et al. Invasive cutaneous squamous cell carcinoma incidence in US health care workers. Arch Dermatol Res 2014;306(6):555–60.

9. Miller DL, Weinstock MA. Nonmelanoma skin cancer in the united states: incidence. J Am Acad Dermatol 1994;30(5 Pt 1):774–8.

10. Stern RS. Prevalence of a history of skin cancer in 2007: results of an incidence-based model. Arch Dermatol 2010;146(3):279–82.

11. Muzic JG, Schmitt AR, Wright AC, et al. Incidence and trends of basal cell carcinoma and cutaneous squamous cell carcinoma: a population-based study in Olmsted County, Minnesota, 2000 to 2010. Mayo Clin Proc 2017;92(6):890–8.

12. Work Group, Invited Reviewers, Kim JYS, Kozlow JH, Mittal B, et al. Guidelines of care for the management of cutaneous squamous cell carcinoma. J Am Acad Dermatol 2018;78(3):560–78.

13. NCCN guidelines in oncology: squamous cell skin cancer. 2018. Available at: https://www.nccn.org/professionals/physician_gls/pdf/squamous.pdf. Accessed July 4, 2018.

14. Allen JE, Stolle LB. Utility of sentinel node biopsy in patients with high-risk cutaneous squamous cell carcinoma. Eur J Surg Oncol 2015;41(2):197–200.

15. Durham AB, Lowe L, Malloy KM, et al. Sentinel lymph node biopsy for cutaneous squamous cell carcinoma on the head and neck. JAMA Otolaryngol Head Neck Surg 2016;142(12):1171–6.

16. Ahadiat O, Higgins S, Sutton A, et al. SLNB in cutaneous SCC: a review of the current state of literature and the direction for the future. J Surg Oncol 2017; 116(3):344–50.

17. Navarrete-Dechent C, Veness MJ, Droppelmann N, et al. High-risk cutaneous squamous cell carcinoma and the emerging role of sentinel lymph node biopsy: a literature review. J Am Acad Dermatol 2015;73(1):127–37.

18. MacFarlane D, Shah K, Wysong A, et al. The role of imaging in the management of patients with nonmelanoma skin cancer: diagnostic modalities and applications. J Am Acad Dermatol 2017;76(4):579–88.

19. Paolino G, Donati M, Didona D, et al. Histology of non-melanoma skin cancers: an update. Biomedicines 2017;5(4) [pii:E71].

20. Murphy G, Beer T, Cerio R, et al. Keratinocytic/epidermal tumors. In: Elder D, Massi D, Scolyer R, et al. World Health Organization classification of Tumours, Fourth Edition. Volume 11. Geneva (Switzerland): WHO Press, World Health Organization. 31–43.

21. Barnard IRM, Tierney P, Campbell CL, et al. Quantifying direct DNA damage in the basal layer of skin exposed to UV radiation from sunbeds. Photochem Photobiol 2018. https://doi.org/10.1111/php.12935.

22. Ikehata H, Mori T, Douki T, et al. Quantitative analysis of UV photolesions suggests that cyclobutane pyrimidine dimers produced in mouse skin by UVB are more mutagenic than those produced by UVC. Photochem Photobiol Sci 2018; 17(4):404–13.

23. Schmitt J, Seidler A, Diepgen TL, et al. Occupational ultraviolet light exposure increases the risk for the development of cutaneous squamous cell carcinoma: a systematic review and meta-analysis. Br J Dermatol 2011;164(2):291–307.
24. Schmitt J, Haufe E, Trautmann F, et al. Is ultraviolet exposure acquired at work the most important risk factor for cutaneous squamous cell carcinoma? Results of the population-based case-control study FB-181. Br J Dermatol 2018;178(2):462–72.
25. Diepgen TL, Fartasch M, Drexler H, et al. Occupational skin cancer induced by ultraviolet radiation and its prevention. Br J Dermatol 2012;167(Suppl 2):76–84.
26. Scotto J, Cotton G, Urbach F, et al. Biologically effective ultraviolet radiation: surface measurements in the United States, 1974 to 1985. Science 1988;239(4841 Pt 1):762–4.
27. Scotto J, Kopf AW, Urbach F. Non-melanoma skin cancer among caucasians in four areas of the United States. Cancer 1974;34(4):1333–8.
28. English DR, Armstrong BK, Kricker A, et al. Case-control study of sun exposure and squamous cell carcinoma of the skin. Int J Cancer 1998;77(3):347–53.
29. Xiang F, Lucas R, Hales S, et al. Incidence of nonmelanoma skin cancer in relation to ambient UV radiation in white populations, 1978-2012: empirical relationships. JAMA Dermatol 2014;150(10):1063–71.
30. Krynitz B, Edgren G, Lindelof B, et al. Risk of skin cancer and other malignancies in kidney, liver, heart and lung transplant recipients 1970 to 2008: a Swedish population-based study. Int J Cancer 2013;132(6):1429–38.
31. Sinnya S, Zwald FO, Colegio OR. Skin cancer in the crosshairs: highlights from the biennial scientific retreat of international transplant skin cancer collaborative and skin care in organ transplant recipients Europe. Transplant Direct 2015;1(7):e26.
32. Zwald FO, Brown M. Skin cancer in solid organ transplant recipients: advances in therapy and management: part II. management of skin cancer in solid organ transplant recipients. J Am Acad Dermatol 2011;65(2):263–79 [quiz: 280].
33. Omland SH, Gniadecki R, Haedersdal M, et al. Skin cancer risk in hematopoietic stem-cell transplant recipients compared with background population and renal transplant recipients: a population-based cohort study. JAMA Dermatol 2016; 152(2):177–83.
34. Velez NF, Karia PS, Vartanov AR, et al. Association of advanced leukemic stage and skin cancer tumor stage with poor skin cancer outcomes in patients with chronic lymphocytic leukemia. JAMA Dermatol 2014;150(3):280–7.
35. Mehrany K, Weenig RH, Lee KK, et al. Increased metastasis and mortality from cutaneous squamous cell carcinoma in patients with chronic lymphocytic leukemia. J Am Acad Dermatol 2005;53(6):1067–71.
36. Mohan SV, Chang J, Li S, et al. Increased risk of cutaneous squamous cell carcinoma after vismodegib therapy for basal cell carcinoma. JAMA Dermatol 2016;152(5):527–32.
37. Faust H, Andersson K, Luostarinen T, et al. Cutaneous human papillomaviruses and squamous cell carcinoma of the skin: nested case-control study. Cancer Epidemiol Biomarkers Prev 2016;25(4):721–4.
38. Torchia D, Massi D, Caproni M, et al. Multiple cutaneous precanceroses and carcinomas from combined iatrogenic/professional exposure to arsenic. Int J Dermatol 2008;47(6):592–3.
39. Balmain A, Yuspa SH. Milestones in skin carcinogenesis: the biology of multistage carcinogenesis. J Invest Dermatol 2014;134(e1):E2–7.
40. Jaju PD, Ransohoff KJ, Tang JY, et al. Familial skin cancer syndromes: increased risk of nonmelanotic skin cancers and extracutaneous tumors. J Am Acad Dermatol 2016;74(3):437–51 [quiz: 452–4].

41. Pickering CR, Zhou JH, Lee JJ, et al. Mutational landscape of aggressive cutaneous squamous cell carcinoma. Clin Cancer Res 2014;20(24):6582–92.

42. Wikonkal NM, Brash DE. Ultraviolet radiation induced signature mutations in photocarcinogenesis. J Investig Dermatol Symp Proc 1999;4(1):6–10.

43. South AP, Purdie KJ, Watt SA, et al. NOTCH1 mutations occur early during cutaneous squamous cell carcinogenesis. J Invest Dermatol 2014;134(10):2630–8.

44. Egashira S, Jinnin M, Ajino M, et al. Chronic sun exposure-related fusion oncogenes EGFR-PPARGC1A in cutaneous squamous cell carcinoma. Sci Rep 2017;7(1):12654.

45. Fears TR, Scotto J. Changes in skin cancer morbidity between 1971-72 and 1977-78. J Natl Cancer Inst 1982;69(2):365–70.

46. Thompson AK, Kelley BF, Prokop LJ, et al. Risk factors for cutaneous squamous cell carcinoma recurrence, metastasis, and disease-specific death: a systematic review and meta-analysis. JAMA Dermatol 2016;152(4):419–28.

47. Karia PS, Jambusaria-Pahlajani A, Harrington DP, et al. Evaluation of American Joint Committee on Cancer, International Union Against Cancer, and Brigham and Women's Hospital tumor staging for cutaneous squamous cell carcinoma. J Clin Oncol 2014;32(4):327–34.

48. Goepfert H, Dichtel WJ, Medina JE, et al. Perineural invasion in squamous cell skin carcinoma of the head and neck. Am J Surg 1984;148(4):542–7.

49. Carter JB, Johnson MM, Chua TL, et al. Outcomes of primary cutaneous squamous cell carcinoma with perineural invasion: an 11-year cohort study. JAMA Dermatol 2013;149(1):35–41.

50. Ross AS, Whalen FM, Elenitsas R, et al. Diameter of involved nerves predicts outcomes in cutaneous squamous cell carcinoma with perineural invasion: an investigator-blinded retrospective cohort study. Dermatol Surg 2009;35(12): 1859–66.

51. Rowe DE, Carroll RJ, Day CL Jr. Prognostic factors for local recurrence, metastasis, and survival rates in squamous cell carcinoma of the skin, ear, and lip. Implications for treatment modality selection. J Am Acad Dermatol 1992;26(6): 976–90.

52. Harris BN, Bayoumi A, Rao S, et al. Factors associated with recurrence and regional adenopathy for head and neck cutaneous squamous cell carcinoma. Otolaryngol Head Neck Surg 2017;156(5):863–9.

53. Wang DM, Kraft S, Rohani P, et al. Association of Nodal Metastasis and Mortality With Vermilion vs Cutaneous Lip Location in Cutaneous Squamous Cell Carcinoma of the Lip. JAMA Dermatol 2018;154(6):701–7.

54. Winkelhorst JT, Brokelman WJ, Tiggeler RG, et al. Incidence and clinical course of de-novo malignancies in renal allograft recipients. Eur J Surg Oncol 2001; 27(4):409–13.

55. Cheng JY, Li FY, Ko CJ, et al. Cutaneous squamous cell carcinomas in solid organ transplant recipients compared with immunocompetent patients. JAMA Dermatol 2018;154(1):60–6.

56. Wheless L, Jacks S, Mooneyham Potter KA, et al. Skin cancer in organ transplant recipients: more than the immune system. J Am Acad Dermatol 2014;71(2): 359–65.

57. Kanitakis J, Karayannopoulou G, Roux A, et al. Histopathologic features predictive of aggressiveness of post-transplant cutaneous squamous-cell carcinomas. Anticancer Res 2015;35(4):2305–8.

58. Garrett GL, Lowenstein SE, Singer JP, et al. Trends of skin cancer mortality after transplantation in the United States: 1987 to 2013. J Am Acad Dermatol 2016; 75(1):106–12.
59. Lam JKS, Sundaresan P, Gebski V, et al. Immunocompromised patients with metastatic cutaneous nodal squamous cell carcinoma of the head and neck: poor outcome unrelated to the index lesion. Head Neck 2018;40(5):985–92.
60. Rizvi SMH, Aagnes B, Holdaas H, et al. Long-term change in the risk of skin cancer after organ transplantation: a population-based nationwide cohort study. JAMA Dermatol 2017;153(12):1270–7.
61. Que SKT, Zwald FO, Schmults CD. Cutaneous squamous cell carcinoma: incidence, risk factors, diagnosis, and staging. J Am Acad Dermatol 2018;78(2): 237–47.
62. Amin M, Edge S, editors. AJCC cancer staging manual. 8th edition. New York: Springer; 2017.
63. Xu MJ, Lazar AA, Garsa AA, et al. Major prognostic factors for recurrence and survival independent of the American Joint Committee on Cancer eighth edition staging system in patients with cutaneous squamous cell carcinoma treated with multimodality therapy. Head Neck 2018;40(7):1406–14.
64. Jambusaria-Pahlajani A, Kanetsky PA, Karia PS, et al. Evaluation of AJCC tumor staging for cutaneous squamous cell carcinoma and a proposed alternative tumor staging system. JAMA Dermatol 2013;149(4):402–10.
65. Lansbury L, Bath-Hextall F, Perkins W, et al. Interventions for non-metastatic squamous cell carcinoma of the skin: systematic review and pooled analysis of observational studies. BMJ 2013;347:f6153.
66. Lansbury L, Leonardi-Bee J, Perkins W, et al. Interventions for non-metastatic squamous cell carcinoma of the skin. Cochrane Database Syst Rev 2010;(4):CD007869.
67. Hirshoren N, Ruskin O, McDowell LJ, et al. Management of parotid metastatic cutaneous squamous cell carcinoma: regional recurrence rates and survival. Otolaryngol Head Neck Surg 2018;159(2):293–9.
68. Navarrete-Dechent C, Veness MJ, Droppelmann N, et al. Cutaneous squamous cell carcinoma and the emerging role of sentinel lymph node biopsy. G Ital Dermatol Venereol 2018;153(3):403–18.
69. Porceddu SV, Bressel M, Poulsen MG, et al. Postoperative concurrent chemoradiotherapy versus postoperative radiotherapy in high-risk cutaneous squamous cell carcinoma of the head and neck: the randomized phase III TROG 05.01 trial. J Clin Oncol 2018;36(13):1275–83.
70. Migden MR, Rischin D, Schmults CD, et al. PD-1 blockade with cemiplimab in advanced cutaneous squamous-cell carcinoma. N Engl J Med 2018;379(4): 341–51.
71. Gold KA, Kies MS, William WN Jr, et al. Erlotinib in the treatment of recurrent or metastatic cutaneous squamous cell carcinoma: a single-arm phase 2 clinical trial. Cancer 2018;124(10):2169–73.
72. Potenza C, Bernardini N, Balduzzi V, et al. A review of the literature of surgical and nonsurgical treatments of invasive squamous cells carcinoma. Biomed Res Int 2018;2018:9489163.
73. Yanagi T, Kitamura S, Hata H. Novel therapeutic targets in cutaneous squamous cell carcinoma. Front Oncol 2018;8:79.
74. Que SKT, Zwald FO, Schmults CD. Cutaneous squamous cell carcinoma: management of advanced and high-stage tumors. J Am Acad Dermatol 2018; 78(2):249–61.

75. van der Pols JC, Williams GM, Pandeya N, et al. Prolonged prevention of squamous cell carcinoma of the skin by regular sunscreen use. Cancer Epidemiol Biomarkers Prev 2006;15(12):2546–8.
76. Olsen CM, Wilson LF, Green AC, et al. Cancers in Australia attributable to exposure to solar ultraviolet radiation and prevented by regular sunscreen use. Aust N Z J Public Health 2015;39(5):471–6.
77. Wheless L, Black J, Alberg AJ. Nonmelanoma skin cancer and the risk of second primary cancers: a systematic review. Cancer Epidemiol Biomarkers Prev 2010; 19(7):1686–95.
78. Song F, Qureshi AA, Giovannucci EL, et al. Risk of a second primary cancer after non-melanoma skin cancer in white men and women: a prospective cohort study. PLoS Med 2013;10(4):e1001433.
79. Wehner MR, Cidre Serrano W, Nosrati A, et al. All-cause mortality in patients with basal and squamous cell carcinoma: a systematic review and meta-analysis. J Am Acad Dermatol 2018;78(4):663–72.e3.
80. Johnson MM, Leachman SA, Aspinwall LG, et al. Skin cancer screening: recommendations for data-driven screening guidelines and a review of the US Preventive Services Task Force controversy. Melanoma Manag 2017;4(1):13–37.
81. Robinson JK, Friedewald J, Gordon EJ. Perceptions of risk of developing skin cancer for diverse audiences: enhancing relevance of sun protection to reduce the risk. J Cancer Educ 2016;31(1):153–7.

Basal Cell Carcinoma Review

Dennis P. Kim, MD[a], Kylee J.B. Kus, BS[b], Emily Ruiz, MD, MPH[c],*

KEYWORDS

- Basal cell carcinoma • BCC • NMSC • Nonmelanoma skin cancer • Mohs • MMS

KEY POINTS

- Basal cell carcinoma (BCC) is the most common malignancy and the incidence and associated costs are rising.
- For superficial tumors or patients who cannot tolerate surgery, topical and nonsurgical methods are available.
- Large or aggressive histologic tumors or those arising in high-risk areas should be treated with Mohs micrographic surgery or excision with complete peripheral and deep margin assessment.
- For locally advanced or metastatic tumors, or patients with a genetic predisposition for BCC, systemic treatment with hedgehog inhibitors may be warranted.

INTRODUCTION

Basal cell carcinoma (BCC) is the most common malignancy and the incidence is rising.[1] BCCs have low mortality but can cause significant morbidity primarily through local destruction.[2] The pathogenesis is linked to the interplay between environmental and patient-derived characteristics. There are multiple therapeutic modalities, and appropriate selection requires knowledge of complications, cosmetic outcomes, and recurrence rates. This article reviews the epidemiology, staging, treatment, and prevention of BCC.

INCIDENCE

BCC is the most common malignancy in the United States and the incidence is increasing by 4% to 8% annually, which is heavily influenced by cumulative sun exposure and an aging population.[1,3] An estimated 5.4 million nonmelanoma skin cancers

Disclosure Statement: The authors have no relevant disclosures.
[a] Mohs Micrographic Surgery, Brigham and Women's Faulkner Hospital, 1153 Centre Street, Suite 4J, Jamaica Plain, MA 02130-3446, USA; [b] Oakland University William Beaumont School of Medicine, 586 Pioneer Drive, Rochester, MI 48309-4482, USA; [c] High-Risk Skin Cancer Clinic, Dana Farber/Brigham and Women's Cancer Center, Mohs and Dermatologic Surgery Center, Brigham and Women's Faulkner Hospital, Harvard Medical School, 1153 Centre Street, Suite 4J, Jamaica Plain, MA 02130-3446, USA
* Corresponding author.
E-mail address: esruiz@bwh.harvard.edu

(NMSCs) were diagnosed in 3.3 million patients in 2012.[4] Despite the high incidence rate, the metastasis and age-adjusted mortality rates are estimated at only 0.0028% to 0.5% and 0.12 per 100,000, respectively.[5] Unpublished data from Brigham and Women's Hospital suggest, however, that the risk of metastasis and death is 6.5% in tumors greater than or equal to 2 cm.[6]

Burden of Disease

From 2007 to 2011, an estimated $4.8 billion was spent on keratinocytic carcinomas annually.[7] In 2013, approximately $715 million was spent on direct BCC care in Medicare beneficiaries.[8] A study estimating both direct (health care, out-of-pocket, and informal caregiver costs), indirect (decreased productivity/output), and intangible (loss of health-related quality of life) costs in 2011 in Canada estimated the total cost per BCC to be $4312.[9]

Pathogenesis

The patched/hedgehog intracellular signaling pathway is responsible for regulating cell growth, and constitutive activation of this pathway leads to BCC development.[10] The most common mutations are inactivating mutations of *PTCH1* or activating mutations of *SMOm*, which cause aberrant hedgehog pathway activation and tumor formation. A loss-of-function mutation in *SUFU*, a negative regulator of the hedgehog pathway, has also been identified in a small portion of BCCs.[11] Other common mutations include UV-specific defects in the *p53* tumor suppressor gene, which are present in half of BCCs.[11]

RISK FACTORS

BCCs are more common in Fitzpatrick skin types I and II, with a lifetime risk estimated at 30%. BCC risk is also associated with light eye color, freckles, and blonde or red hair.[1] UV radiation exposure is the most important environmental risk factor. Other risk factors include childhood sunburns, family history of skin cancer, tanning bed use, chronic immunosuppression, photosensitizing drugs, ionizing radiation, and exposure to carcinogenic chemicals, especially arsenic.[1,12–15] Childhood and intense and intermittent sun exposure has a strong correlation to BCC development.[12,16]

Immunosuppression

The estimated incidence of BCC is double in HIV-positive patients and 5-times to 10-times greater in organ transplant patients.[17] Approximately half of organ transplant recipients develop a BCC during the 10 years after transplant and tumors are more likely to be the thinner, superficial histologic subtype and occur in younger patients.[18] Methotrexate use in patients with rheumatoid or psoriatic arthritis has been shown to have a dose-response relationship with BCC incidence.[19]

Genetic Syndromes

Multiple BCCs is the hallmark of basal cell nevus syndrome (BCNS).[20] BCNS is caused by loss of *PTCH1* protein function. This defect causes constitutive activation of hedgehog signaling and tumor cell proliferation.[21] Although most cases of BCNS are inherited in an autosomal dominant manner, approximately 26% to 50% of cases are de novo.[21] Xeroderma pigmentosums a rare autosomal recessive disorder due to defects in nucleotide excision repair pathway proteins. BCC is the most common malignancy and typically diagnosed in the first decade of life.[22] Bazex-Dupre-Christol syndrome is a rare X-linked dominant disorder that presents with follicular atrophoderma, hypohidrosis, hypotrichosis, milia, and multiple facial BCCs that first appear in the third and fourth decades.[23]

HISTOLOGIC SUBTYPES

Lower-risk histologic subtypes[24–26]:

- Superficial BCC is an indolent variant that often has a multifocal pattern. Lesions are pink, scaly, thin plaques that can mimic eczema or psoriasis.
- Nodular BCCs are the most common variant. Tumors present as well-defined, pearly, translucent papules or nodules with rolled borders and telangiectasias. Dermoscopy shows arborizing vessels, large blue-gray ovoid nests, and multiple blue-gray dots.
- Pigmented BCC is a subtype of nodular BCC that is more common in individuals with Fitzpatrick skin types III to VI. Dermoscopy can highlight the pigment globules, which help differentiate pigmented BCCs from melanocytic lesions.

Higher-risk histologic subtypes[26–28]:

- Morpheaform (sclerosing) BCCs have higher rates of recurrence and perineural invasion. Tumors present as a depressed, waxy, scarlike plaques, often accompanied by ulceration.
- Infiltrative BCC is associated with higher rates of perineural invasion and recurrence.
- Micronodular BCCs are composed of dispersed micronodules whereas nodular BCCs are composed of aggregated nodules.
- Basosquamous carcinoma behaves more similarly to squamous cell carcinoma (SCC). Basosquamous carcinoma histologically consists of BCC and SCC in different areas with a transition zone of mixed differentiation, distinguishing this tumor from collision tumors.

GRADING AND STAGING

There is no formal BCC staging system. Prior to the seventh edition of the American Joint Committee on Cancer (AJCC), BCC staging was grouped with all NMSC. The AJCC seventh edition created a distinct staging system for SCC that excluded BCCs. The most useful stratification framework is provided by the National Comprehensive Cancer Network (NCCN), which differentiates localized tumors at low-risk versus high-risk for recurrence.

Clinical Factors

Anatomic location is a known risk factor for BCC recurrence. The appropriate use criteria for Mohs micrographic surgery (MMS) and NCCN guidelines designate 3 body areas for risk stratification based on primary tumor location. Area H is considered the high-risk location, independent of tumor size. Tumors arising in the M and L areas can be classified as high risk, depending on the size, histologic subtype, and poorly defined borders. BCCs developing in the setting of immunosuppression and recurrent tumors, irrespective of prior therapy, are also considered high-risk.[24,26]

Pathologic Factors

Micronodular, infiltrative, sclerosing, and morpheaform histologic subtypes are more likely to recur than nodular or superficial BCCs.[29] Perineural involvement (PNI) is rare with an incidence of less than 1% but is an independent risk factor for recurrence and is more common with aggressive subtypes.[30] One prospective multicenter case series found the 5-year recurrence rate of BCCs with PNI after MMS to be 7.7%.[30] MRI should be considered to evaluate nerve involvement if patients exhibit neurologic symptoms.

New Classification System

Data from the unpublished Brigham and Women's Hospital cohort found that head and neck location (odds ratio [OR] 5.3; 95% CI, 1.2–23.2), depth beyond fat (OR 28.6; 95% CI, 6.7–121), and tumor diameter greater than or equal to 4 cm (OR 11.9; 95% CI, 2.4–59.4) were significant predictors of metastasis and death.[6] A T classification system (T1, T2, and T3) has been developed based on these characteristics. T3 tumors are greater than or equal to 2 cm and contained at least 2 of the 3 high-risk factors. The 10-year cumulative incidence rates of local recurrence and metastasis or death were 47% (95% CI, 28%–70%) and 37% (95% CI, 21%–60%), respectively, in this cohort.

TREATMENT

BCC treatment is primarily directed at local control given its low metastatic potential. When comparing the cure rates for treatments based on different studies, several factors should be considered, including the duration of follow-up and the percentage of high-risk and recurrent tumors. For example, due to the slow growth rate of BCCs, recurrences are often diagnosed after 5 years.[31] The recurrence rate in a randomized controlled trial (RCT) of surgical excision was 3% and 12% at 2.5 years and 10 years, respectively, and 56% of recurrences occurred more than 5 years post-treatment.[32]

Surgical Excision

The NCCN recommends 4-mm clinical margins for low-risk tumors treated with standard excision with postoperative margin assessment (SEPMA).[33] Primary tumors of any size on the neck, trunk, and extremities have in excess of 95% 5-year cure rate.[34] Rates of incomplete excisions are estimated at 3% to 16.6% and are associated with a recurrence rate of approximately 38%.[35] Surgical excision is less effective for BCCs arising in the H-area possibly due to narrower margins used, more aggressive histology, or increased subclinical spread.[36]

Mohs Micrographic Surgery

MMS has superior long-term cure rates compared with other treatment modalities and is the treatment of choice for high-risk and recurrent BCCs. The 5-year recurrence rates for primary and recurrent BCCs treated with MMS are 1% and 5.6%, respectively, compared with 10.1% and 17.4%, respectively, for SEPMA.[37] The 10-year recurrence rates in the only RCT comparing MMS with SEPMA for primary facial BCCs were 4.4% for MMS and 12.2% for SEPMA ($P = .10$) for primary BCCs.[32] For recurrent BCCs, the 10-year recurrence rates were 3.9% and 13.5% ($P = .023$) for MMS and SEPMA, respectively.[32] The high cure rate is due to the complete peripheral and deep margin assessment (CCPDMA), where approximately 100% of the margin is assessed, whereas standard vertical sectioning evaluates approximately 1% of the margins.[38] In 2012, the appropriate use criteria for MMS were released and guidelines for BCC are summarized in **Table 1**.[26]

Table 1
Appropriate use criteria for treatment of basal cell carcinoma with Mohs micrographic surgery

Basal Cell Carcinoma Subtype	Area H	Area M	Area L
Primary superficial BCC	Appropriate	Appropriate • If ≥0.6 cm for non-IC • Any size if IC	Not indicated[a]
Primary nodular BCC	Appropriate	Appropriate	Appropriate • If >1 cm for non-IC • If >2 cm IC
Primary high-risk BCC	Appropriate	Appropriate	Appropriate[a] • If >0.5 cm
Recurrent BCC	Appropriate	Appropriate	Appropriate (except for superficial subtype)[a]

Abbreviation: IC, immunocompromised.

[a] Mohs surgery is indicated, regardless of lesion size or superficial histology, under special clinical circumstances, including previously irradiated field, genetic syndromes, chronic ulcer or inflammation, and traumatic scar.

Adapted from Connolly SM, Baker DR, Coldiron BM, et al. AAD/ACMS/ASDSA/ASMS 2012 appropriate use criteria for Mohs micrographic surgery: a report of the American Academy of Dermatology, American College of Mohs Surgery, American Society for Dermatologic Surgery Association, and the American Society for Mohs Surgery. J Am Acad Dermatol 2012;67(4):542; with permission.

Curettage and Electrodessication

Curettage and electrodessication (CE) is recommended by the NCCN for properly selected, low-risk tumors. CE is fast and cost-effective; however, it does not allow for histologic margin assessment and is operator-dependent.[39] Areas with terminal hair growth should be avoided due to the risk of follicular tumor extension. Larger lesion diameter and high-risk anatomic sites have been shown to be independent factors for recurrence. A study of more than 2300 BCCs found a 5-year recurrence rate of 3.3% (standard error [SE] = 1.5%) for lesions of any diameter treated in the L area. For tumors in the M area, the 5-year recurrence rates were 5.3% (SE = 2.7%) and 22.7% (SE = 7.2%) for BCCs with diameters of less than 10 mm or greater than 10 mm, respectively. For BCCs in the H area, the 5-year recurrence rates were 4.5% (SE ≤ 2.6%) and 17.6% (SE ≤ 5.4%) for tumors less than 6 mm or greater than 6 mm, respectively.[40] Patients treated with CE have reported worse cosmetic outcomes compared with MMS.[41]

Cryosurgery

Cryosurgery is a fast, destructive technique but lacks histologic assessment of tumor margin. The goal is to achieve −50°C to the tumor with a surrounding margin of 3 mm to 5 mm. Although multiple large case series report cures rates of 94% to 99%, careful patient and tumor selection is essential and should be reserved to superficial and low-risk tumors.[42]

Photodynamic Therapy

Photodynamic therapy (PDT) with aminolevulinic acid (ALA) and methyl aminolevulinate (MAL) have similar outcomes and pain scores when used to treat nodular BCC.[43] Cure rates range from 70% to 90%, although approximately all studies have short follow-up periods.[44,45] The 5-year recurrence rates in an RCT were 30.7%

(95% CI, 21.5%–42.6%) for ALA-PDT and 2.3% (95% CI, 0.6%%–8.8%) for surgical excision ($P < .0001$). When stratified by tumor thickness, however, the ALA-PDT cure rate approached 95% for primary thin nodular BCCs ($\leq$0.7-mm thick).[46] PDT should be considered for patients with superficial BCCs, in particular those with extensive/multifocal disease or diffuse actinic damage.

Radiation

Radiation therapy (RT) can be considered a primary therapy in patients for whom surgery is contraindicated or for tumors that are unresectable. The NCCN recommends adjuvant RT for any BCC with large caliber or extensive PNI.[24] RT is generally reserved for patients over 60 years of age and is contraindicated in patients with predisposing genetic syndromes, such as BCNS, due to their risk of other ionizing radiation-induced malignancies.[47] Retrospective studies report 5-year recurrence rates up to 27.7% for BCCs.[48] RT tends to be more effective for treating tumors that are primary (vs recurrent), less than 1 cm, and have less aggressive histologic subtypes.[49,50] RT is also associated with poorer cosmetic outcomes and more postoperative complications.[51]

Topical Therapies

Imiquimod and fluorouracil creams are approved by the US Food and Drug Administration (FDA) to treat superficial BCCs. The recommended treatment regimen for imiquimod is a once-daily application 5 days per week for 6 weeks to 12 weeks and has been associated with up to 81% cure rates.[52] An RCT comparing the efficacy of imiquimod, fluorouracil, and MAL-PDT for the treatment of superficial BCC found that at 3 years, imiquimod (tumor-free survival: 79.7%; 95% CI, 71.6%–85.7%) was superior to MAL-PDT (tumor free survival: 58.0%; 95% CI, 47.8%–66.9%) and fluorouracil (tumor-free survival: 68.2%, 95% CI, 58.1%–76.3%).[53] Topical therapies are associated with adverse side effects, including erythema, swelling, and erosions, which can limit compliance and decrease effectiveness. Use should be limited to superficial BCCs and small tumors in low-risk locations that cannot undergo treatment with more definitive therapies.[52]

Systemic Therapies

Although a majority of BCCs are easily cured with local treatment, a subset of patients, including those with BCNS and locally advanced or metastatic disease, require systemic treatment. In 2012, the FDA approved vismodegib, a first-in-class hedgehog pathway inhibitor, for the treatment of locally advanced or metastatic BCCs.[54] Approval was granted based on the clinical efficacy demonstrated in the ERIVANCE phase 2 study (**Tables 2** and **3**).[55] Objective responses of 48% and 33% for patients with locally advanced and metastatic disease, respectively, were reported at 21-month follow-up.[56] Nearly all patients treated with vismodegib experienced at least 1 adverse effect, including muscle spasms, alopecia, dysgeusia, weight loss, fatigue, or diarrhea. Grade 3 or 4 adverse effects occurred in 25% of patients.[57] A double-blind randomized phase 2 study of patients with BCNS found that vismodegib significantly reduced the incidence of new BCCs and the size of existing tumors. Unfortunately, only 17% of patients tolerated vismodegib continuously for the full 36-month study duration. Vismodegib can be taken with or without food and does not require laboratory work prior to or after initiation.[54] There are reports, however, of hepatotoxicity, so caution should be taken in patients with severe liver disease.[58]

Sonidegib, the second hedgehog pathway inhibitor, is approved by the FDA for treatment of locally advanced BCCs that recur after surgery or RT or who are not candidates for surgery or radiotherapy. The phase 2 Basal Cell Carcinoma Outcomes with

Table 2
Efficacy of sonidegib and vismodegib in patients with locally advanced basal cell carcinoma

| | Sonidegib, 200 mg | Vismodegib, 150 mg | | |
	BOLT 12-mo Analysis	ERIVANCE 21-mo Analysis	Vismodegib Expanded Access	STEVIE
Minimum follow-up	12	21	Not reported	12
Patients, n	42	71	56	453
Objective response rate	43%	48%	46%	67%
Time to response, median	3.9	Not reported	2.6	2.6
Duration response, median	Not reached	9.5	Not reported	22.7
Progression free survival, median months (% progressed)	Not reached (12%)	9.5 (3%)	Not reported (0%)	24.5 (2%)

Times are reported in months.
Abbreviation: STEVIE study, Safety Events in Vismodegib.
Data from Refs.[56,59,66,67]

LDE225 Treatment (BOLT) trial found response rates of 44% to 58% for locally advanced BCC and 8% to 17% for metastatic BCC (see **Tables 2** and **3**).[59] Nearly all patients experienced at least 1 adverse effect with elevated creatinine kinase and lipase the most common grade 3 or grade 4 adverse effects. Sonidegib should be taken on an empty stomach and should not be administered concomitantly with strong and moderate CYP3A inhibitors.[60]

Two main limitations to hedgehog pathway inhibitor therapy are the high frequency of adverse effects and development of tumor resistance. Intermittent dosing regimens have been trialed as a way to minimize side effects while not compromising efficacy.[61] Patients with BCNS respond to vismodegib and have a low acquired resistance.[62] Advanced and metastatic BCC patients, however, have lower overall response rates (approximately 48%) and an estimated 20% develop resistance during their first year.[63]

Table 3
Efficacy of sonidegib and vismodegib in patients with metastatic basal cell carcinoma

| | Sonidegib, 200 mg | Vismodegib, 150 mg | | |
	BOLT 12-mo Analysis	ERIVANCE 21-mo Analysis	Vismodegib Expanded Access	STEVIE
Minimum follow-up	12	21	Not reported	12
Patients, n	13	33	39	29
Objective response rate	15%	33%	31%	38%
Time to response, median	4.6	Not reported	2.6	2.8
Duration response, median	Not reached	7.6	Not reported	10
Progression free survival, median months (% progressed)	13.1 (31%)	9.5 (13%)	Not reported (8%)	13.1 (14%)

Times are reported in months.
Abbreviation: STEVIE, Safety Events in Vismodegib.
Data from Refs.[56,59,66]

Anti–programmed death-1 (PD-1) immunotherapy is another emerging treatment option for advanced BCC. A clinical trial investigating cemiplimab, a fully human anti–PD-1 monoclonal antibody, in patients with locally advanced or metastatic BCC who experienced progression of disease or stable disease on or who cannot tolerate hedgehog pathway inhibitor therapy is under way.

FOLLOW-UP AND PREVENTION

Patients with a history of BCC are at risk for additional skin cancers, including NMSC and melanoma.[64] A prospective cohort study of 1426 patients found the risk for subsequent NMSC to be 40.7% (95% CI, 36.5%–45.2%) after a first and 82% (95% CI, 80.2%–83.7%) after more than 1 NMSC at 5 years.[64] Thus, continued long-term surveillance of patients with a history of BCC is essential. The NCCN recommends skin examinations at least every 6 months to 12 months for the first 2 years after BCC diagnosis and then reduced to annually if appropriate.[24] Patients also should be educated about UV protection.[65]

SUMMARY

BCC is a slowly growing tumor that can generally be cured easily with office-based surgical methods. For superficial tumors or patients who cannot tolerate surgery, topical and nonsurgical methods are available. Large or aggressive histologic tumors or those arising in high-risk areas should be treated with MMS or excision with CCPDMA. For locally advanced or metastatic tumors, or in patients with a genetic predisposition for BCC, systemic treatment with hedgehog inhibitors may be warranted. Close follow-up for early diagnosis and treatment of subsequent BCCs is essential.

REFERENCES

1. Lai V, Cranwell W, Sinclair R. Epidemiology of skin cancer in the mature patient. Clin Dermatol 2018;36(2):167–76.
2. Kasper M, Jaks V, Hohl D, et al. Basal cell carcinoma - molecular biology and potential new therapies. J Clin Invest 2012;122(2):455–63.
3. Cameron MC, Lee E, Hibler B, et al. Basal cell carcinoma: part 1. J Am Acad Dermatol 2018 [pii:S0190-9622(18)30775-8].
4. Rogers HW, Weinstock MA, Feldman SR, et al. Incidence estimate of nonmelanoma skin cancer (Keratinocyte Carcinomas) in the US Population, 2012. JAMA Dermatol 2015;151(10):1081.
5. von Domarus H, Stevens PJ. Metastatic basal cell carcinoma. Report of five cases and review of 170 cases in the literature. J Am Acad Dermatol 1984; 10(6):1043–60.
6. Morgan FC, Ruiz ES, Karia PS. Factors predictive of recurrence, metastasis, and death from primary basal cell carcinoma 2cm or larger in diameter. in press.
7. Guy GP, Machlin SR, Ekwueme DU, et al. Prevalence and costs of skin cancer treatment in the U.S., 2002-2006 and 2007-2011. Am J Prev Med 2015;48(2): 183–7.
8. Ruiz ES, Morgan FC, Zigler CM, et al. National skin cancer expenditure analysis in the United States medicare population, 2013. J Am Acad Dermatol 2018. [Epub ahead of print].
9. Mofidi A, Tompa E, Spencer J, et al. The economic burden of occupational nonmelanoma skin cancer due to solar radiation. J Occup Environ Hyg 2018;15(6): 481–91.

10. Sehgal VN, Chatterjee K, Pandhi D, et al. Basal cell carcinoma: pathophysiology. Skinmed 2014;12(3):176–81.

11. Bonilla X, Parmentier L, King B, et al. Genomic analysis identifies new drivers and progression pathways in skin basal cell carcinoma. Nat Genet 2016;48(4): 398–406.

12. Gallagher RP, Hill GB, Bajdik CD, et al. Sunlight exposure, pigmentary factors, and risk of nonmelanocytic skin cancer. Arch Dermatol 1995;131(2):157.

13. Robinson SN, Zens MS, Perry AE, et al. Photosensitizing agents and the risk of non-melanoma skin cancer: a population-based case–control study. J Invest Dermatol 2013;133(8):1950–5.

14. Karagas MR, McDonald JA, Greendberg ER, et al. Risk of basal cell and squamous cell skin cancers after ionizing radiation therapy. J Natl Cancer Inst 1996; 88(24):1848–53.

15. Martinez VD, Vucic EA, Becker-Santos DD, et al. Arsenic exposure and the induction of human cancers. J Toxicol 2011;2011:431287.

16. Kricker A, Armstrong BK, English DR, et al. Does intermittent sun exposure cause basal cell carcinoma? a case-control study in Western Australia. Int J Cancer 1995;60(4):489–94.

17. Silverberg MJ, Leyden W, Warton EM, et al. HIV infection status, immunodeficiency, and the incidence of non-melanoma skin cancer. J Natl Cancer Inst 2013;105(5):350–60.

18. Harwood CA, Proby CM, McGregor JM, et al. Clinicopathologic features of skin cancer in organ transplant recipients: a retrospective case-control series. J Am Acad Dermatol 2006;54(2):290–300.

19. Lange E, Blizzard L, Venn A, et al. Disease-modifying anti-rheumatic drugs and non-melanoma skin cancer in inflammatory arthritis patients: a retrospective cohort study. Rheumatology 2016;55(9):1594–600.

20. Bresler SC, Padwa BL, Granter SR. Nevoid basal cell carcinoma syndrome (Gorlin Syndrome). Head Neck Pathol 2016;10(2):119–24.

21. Akbari M, Chen H, Guo G, et al. Basal cell nevus syndrome (Gorlin syndrome): genetic insights, diagnostic challenges, and unmet milestones. Pathophysiology 2018;25(2):77–82.

22. DiGiovanna JJ, Kraemer KH. Shining a light on xeroderma pigmentosum. J Invest Dermatol 2012;132(3 Pt 2):785–96.

23. AlSabbagh MM, Baqi MA. Bazex-Dupré-Christol syndrome: review of clinical and molecular aspects. Int J Dermatol 2018;57(9):1102–6.

24. Bichakjian CK. NCCN guidelines version 1.2018 basal cell skin cancer. NCCN Guidel. 2018. Available at: www.nccn.org. Accessed July 15, 2018.

25. Saldanha G, Fletcher A, Slater DN. Basal cell carcinoma: a dermatopathological and molecular biological update. Br J Dermatol 2003;148(2):195–202.

26. Connolly SM, Baker DR, Coldiron BM, et al. AAD/ACMS/ASDSA/ASMS 2012 appropriate use criteria for Mohs micrographic surgery: a report of the American Academy of Dermatology, American College of Mohs Surgery, American Society for Dermatologic Surgery Association, and the American Society for Mohs Surgery. J Am Acad Dermatol 2012;67(4):531–50.

27. Hendrix JD, Parlette HL. Micronodular basal cell carcinoma. Arch Dermatol 1996; 132(3):295.

28. Akay BN, Saral S, Heper AO, et al. Basosquamous carcinoma: dermoscopic clues to diagnosis. J Dermatol 2017;44(2):127–34.

29. Szewczyk MP, Pazdrowski J, Dańczak-Pazdrowska A, et al. Analysis of selected recurrence risk factors after treatment of head and neck basal cell carcinoma. Postepy Dermatol Allergol 2014;31(3):146–51.

30. Leibovitch I, Huilgol SC, Selva D, et al. Basal cell carcinoma treated with Mohs surgery in Australia III. Perineural invasion. J Am Acad Dermatol 2005;53(3): 458–63.

31. Rowe DE. Comparison of treatment modalities for basal cell carcinoma. Clin Dermatol 1995;13(6):617–20.

32. van Loo E, Mosterd K, Krekels GAM, et al. Surgical excision versus Mohs' micrographic surgery for basal cell carcinoma of the face: a randomised clinical trial with 10 year follow-up. Eur J Cancer 2014;50(17):3011–20.

33. Fields RC, Fleming MD, Gastman B, et al. NCCN Clinical Practice Guidelines in Oncology (NCCN Guidelines®) Melanoma - Version 2.2018. 2018.

34. Codazzi D, Van Der Velden J, Carminati M, et al. Positive compared with negative margins in a single-centre retrospective study on 3957 consecutive excisions of basal cell carcinomas. Associated risk factors and preferred surgical management. J Plast Surg Hand Surg 2014;48(1):38–43.

35. Sherry KR, Reid LA, Wilmshurst AD. A five year review of basal cell carcinoma excisions. J Plast Reconstr Aesthet Surg 2010;63(9):1485–9.

36. Kjerkegaard UK, Stolle LB. Incomplete excision of non-melanoma skin cancer of the head and neck: can we predict failure? Eur J Plast Surg 2014;37(3):141–6.

37. Rowe DE, Carroll RJ, Day CL. Mohs surgery is the treatment of choice for recurrent (previously treated) basal cell carcinoma. J Dermatol Surg Oncol 1989;15(4): 424–31.

38. Abide JM, Nahai F, Bennett RG. The meaning of surgical margins. Plast Reconstr Surg 1984;73(3):492–7.

39. Goldman G. The current status of curettage and electrodesiccation. Dermatol Clin 2002;20(3):569–78, ix.

40. Silverman MK, Kopf AW, Grin CM, et al. Recurrence rates of treated basal cell carcinomas. Part 2: curettage-electrodesiccation. J Dermatol Surg Oncol 1991; 17(9):720–6.

41. Galles E, Parvataneni R, Stuart SE, et al. Patient-reported outcomes of electrodessication and curettage for treatment of nonmelanoma skin cancer. J Am Acad Dermatol 2014;71(5):1026–8.

42. Kuflik EG. Cryosurgery for skin cancer: 30-year experience and cure rates. Dermatol Surg 2004;30(2 Pt 2):297–300.

43. Kuijpers DI, Thissen MR, Thissen CA, et al. Similar effectiveness of methyl aminolevulinate and 5-aminolevulinate in topical photodynamic therapy for nodular basal cell carcinoma. J Drugs Dermatol 2006;5(7):642–5.

44. Savoia P, Deboli T, Previgliano A, et al. Usefulness of photodynamic therapy as a possible therapeutic alternative in the treatment of basal cell carcinoma. Int J Mol Sci 2015;16(10):23300–17.

45. Stebbins WG, Hanke CW. MAL-PDT for difficult to treat nonmelanoma skin cancer. Dermatol Ther 2011;24(1):82–93.

46. Roozeboom MH, Aardoom MA, Nelemans PJ, et al. Fractionated 5-aminolevulinic acid photodynamic therapy after partial debulking versus surgical excision for nodular basal cell carcinoma: a randomized controlled trial with at least 5-year follow-up. J Am Acad Dermatol 2013;69(2):280–7.

47. Neville JA, Welch E, Leffell DJ. Management of nonmelanoma skin cancer in 2007. Nat Clin Pract Oncol 2007;4(8):462–9.

48. Zagrodnik B, Kempf W, Seifert B, et al. Superficial radiotherapy for patients with basal cell carcinoma. Cancer 2003;98(12):2708–14.
49. Wilder RB, Shimm DS, Kittelson JM, et al. Recurrent basal cell carcinoma treated with radiation therapy. Arch Dermatol 1991;127(11):1668–72.
50. Silverman MK, Kopf AW, Gladstein AH, et al. Recurrence rates of treated basal cell carcinomas. Part 4: X-ray therapy. J Dermatol Surg Oncol 1992;18(7):549–54.
51. Petit JY, Avril MF, Margulis A, et al. Evaluation of cosmetic results of a randomized trial comparing surgery and radiotherapy in the treatment of basal cell carcinoma of the face. Plast Reconstr Surg 2000;105(7):2544–51.
52. Love WE, Bernhard JD, Bordeaux JS. Topical imiquimod or fluorouracil therapy for basal and squamous cell carcinoma: a systematic review. Arch Dermatol 2009;145(12):1431–8.
53. Roozeboom MH, Arits AHMM, Mosterd K, et al. Three-year follow-up results of photodynamic therapy vs. imiquimod vs. Fluorouracil for treatment of superficial basal cell carcinoma: a single-blind, noninferiority, randomized controlled trial. J Invest Dermatol 2016;136(8):1568–74.
54. Erivedge (vismodegib) [US prescribing information]. South San Francisco (CA): Genentech Inc; 2012.
55. Sekulic A, Migden MR, Oro AE, et al. Efficacy and safety of vismodegib in advanced basal-cell carcinoma. N Engl J Med 2012;366(23):2171–9.
56. Sekulic A, Migden MR, Lewis K, et al. Pivotal ERIVANCE basal cell carcinoma (BCC) study: 12-month update of efficacy and safety of vismodegib in advanced BCC. J Am Acad Dermatol 2015;72(6):1021–6.e8.
57. Basset-Séguin N, Hauschild A, Kunstfeld R, et al. Vismodegib in patients with advanced basal cell carcinoma: primary analysis of STEVIE, an international, open-label trial. Eur J Cancer 2017;86:334–48.
58. Edwards BJ, Raisch DW, Saraykar SS, et al. Hepatotoxicity with vismodegib: an MD Anderson Cancer Center and Research on adverse drug events and reports project. Drugs R D 2017;17(1):211–8.
59. Lear JT, Migden MR, Lewis KD, et al. Long-term efficacy and safety of sonidegib in patients with locally advanced and metastatic basal cell carcinoma: 30-month analysis of the randomized phase 2 BOLT study. J Eur Acad Dermatol Venereol 2018;32(3):372–81.
60. Novartis. Odomzo® (sonidegib) capsules, for oral use: US prescribing information. Accessed June 27, 2018.
61. Dréno B, Kunstfeld R, Hauschild A, et al. Two intermittent vismodegib dosing regimens in patients with multiple basal-cell carcinomas (MIKIE): a randomised, regimen-controlled, double-blind, phase 2 trial. Lancet Oncol 2017;18(3):404–12. Available at: www.thelancet.com/oncology.
62. Tang JY, Mackay-Wiggan JM, Aszterbaum M, et al. Inhibiting the hedgehog pathway in patients with the basal-cell nevus syndrome. N Engl J Med 2012;366(23):2180–8.
63. Chang ALS, Oro AE. Initial assessment of tumor regrowth after vismodegib in advanced basal cell carcinoma. Arch Dermatol 2012;148(11):1324.
64. Wehner MR, Linos E, Parvataneni R, et al. Timing of subsequent new tumors in patients who present with basal cell carcinoma or cutaneous squamous cell carcinoma. JAMA Dermatol 2015;151(4):382.
65. Veierød MB, Couto E, Lund E, et al. Host characteristics, sun exposure, indoor tanning and risk of squamous cell carcinoma of the skin. Int J Cancer 2014;135(2):413–22.

66. Chang ALS, Solomon JA, Hainsworth JD, et al. Expanded access study of patients with advanced basal cell carcinoma treated with the Hedgehog pathway inhibitor, vismodegib. J Am Acad Dermatol 2014;70(1):60–9.
67. Tilley C, Deep G, Agarwal R. Chemopreventive opportunities to control basal cell carcinoma: current perspectives. Mol Carcinog 2015;54(9):688–97.

Cutaneous Melanoma—A Review in Detection, Staging, and Management

Rebecca I. Hartman, MD, MPH[a,b], Jennifer Y. Lin, MD[a,b],*

KEYWORDS

- Melanoma • Malignant melanoma • Cutaneous melanoma • Immunotherapy
- Targeted therapy • Sentinel lymph node biopsy

KEY POINTS

- Melanoma is an increasingly common cancer in the United States that is highly curable with low morbidity local, surgery alone if diagnosed early, although there is insufficient evidence for routine screening.
- Advances in immunotherapy and targeted therapy over the past decade have dramatically changed treatment paradigms and improved the prognosis for advanced-staged disease.
- In the future, promising advances in diagnostic accuracy via technological improvements and in staging via molecular markers will likely further improve the ability to diagnose and treat melanoma and further enhance its prognosis.

INTRODUCTION

Melanoma, a tumor arising from a melanocyte (the cell responsible for producing pigment), continues to carry the potential to be a deadly disease. In the United States, 91,320 new cases are predicted to be diagnosed in the year 2018, continuing a long-standing trend of rising incidence since 1975.[1] Cutaneous melanoma (CM) is the leading cause of death from skin cancer, with 9320 deaths predicted in 2018.[1] Although 5-year melanoma-specific mortality rates are relatively low, at 8.2%, the spectra of melanoma looms large.[1] It is the eighth most common cause of cancer death in Australia,[2] and in young adults (15–29 years old) living in the United States, it is the second most commonly diagnosed cancer.[3]

Although the rise in incidence likely points to improved detection, the lack of a corresponding drop in mortality has led to concern that the detected CMs were not reliably destined to be lethal and that much work remained to improve earlier detection of

Disclosure Statement: No disclosures.
a Department of Dermatology, Brigham and Women's Hospital, 41 Avenue Louis Pasteur, Room 319, Boston, MA 02115, USA; b Melanoma Program, Dana-Farber Cancer Institute, 450 Brookline Avenue, Boston, MA 02115, USA
* Corresponding author. 41 Avenue Louis Pasteur, Room 219, Boston, MA 02115.
E-mail address: jlin@bwh.harvard.edu

Hematol Oncol Clin N Am 33 (2019) 25–38
https://doi.org/10.1016/j.hoc.2018.09.005
0889-8588/19/© 2018 Elsevier Inc. All rights reserved.

hemonc.theclinics.com

deadly melanomas. There recently has been, however, a stabilization of melanoma mortality in the United States.[4]

Melanoma has also been the tumor to watch in the past decade because of advances in the treatment of metastatic disease. Breakthroughs in immunotherapy that are relevant to melanoma biology have paved the way for treatment of other cancers. In addition, significant changes in pathologic staging and surgical management are all worth noting.

This review provides an evidence-based overview on the detection and staging of melanoma as well as a brief review of the current surgical and medical management. A deeper look into the nuances of the medical management of metastatic melanoma is beyond the scope of this review. The authors highlight the areas where questions remain and end with a discussion on prevention strategies.

DIAGNOSIS AND DETECTION

CM as highly curable if detected early. There are numerous established risk factors, with age and white race the 2 most obvious from US epidemiologic data (**Box 1**).[1] Indoor tanning,[5] classified as a carcinogen by the World Health Organization,[6] is also a risk factor, especially in young women. Most risk factors individually confer a small increased risk, except genetic syndromes, such as familial malignant melanoma (CDKN2a mutation), which is also associated with pancreatic cancer.[7] Although the vast majority (more than 90%) of melanoma is cutaneous, it can initially present as ocular, mucosal, and of unknown primary.[8]

Although physician-detected CMs are thinner than patient-detected,[9] the US Preventive Service Task Force has found insufficient evidence for routine skin cancer screening, by either patients or health care providers.[10] The largest screening study to date is an observational nationwide skin cancer screening program in Germany by general practitioners that found no change in melanoma-specific mortality.[11]

CM is initially diagnosed via visual skin inspection. Diagnostic clues include asymmetry, border, color, diameter, and evolution (ABCDEs) and the ugly duckling sign[12] (**Fig. 1**). Importantly, use of dermoscopy by experienced providers can improve diagnostic accuracy.[13] Additionally, several new technologies seek to improve prebiopsy

---

Box 1
Risk factors for melanoma development

Male gender

Increasing age

Family history of melanoma

Dysplastic (atypical) nevus

Multiple ($\geq$100) nevi

Fair complexion

History of sunburns

Indoor tanning use

History of skin cancer

Data from Final recommendation statement: skin cancer: screening. U.S. preventive services task force. 2016. Available at: https://www.uspreventiveservicestaskforce.org/Page/Document/RecommendationStatementFinal/skin-cancer-screening2. Accessed August 29, 2018.

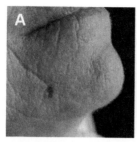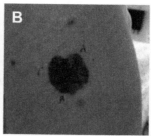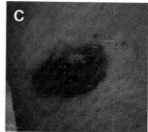

Fig. 1. Clinical photos of CM; most CM evolve over time. (*A*) Melanoma in situ on sun-damaged skin can exhibit few features except for irregularity of pigmentation and early dermoscopy signs. (*B*) T1 melanomas can develop a prominent radial growth phase, initially growing outward, but careful examination demonstrates gray stippling in the area marked "C" as evidence of early invasion. (*C*) Late-stage tumors, such as this T3 lesion, have developed a vertical growth phase and developed a nodule in this preexisting nevus. Vertical growth phase and nodular components of melanomas can grow rapidly and are more likely to be amelanotic.

diagnostic accuracy. These include artificial intelligence image analysis, whole-body 3-D imaging, reflectance confocal microscopy (RCM), optical coherence tomography (OCT), and epidermal genetic information retrieval from adhesive tape stripping. Although they offer potential advantages, none at present is used regularly clinically except for digital photographic monitoring. CMs detected by whole-body photography and sequential digital dermoscopy are thinner than those detected by conventional means.[14] Increasingly, RCM and OCT are used in conjunction with other data points, for instance, to determine the borders of lentigo maligna (LM) in vivo.[15] As the technology becomes more facile and accessible, RCM and OCT will likely be used increasingly in the future.

A diagnosis of CM is confirmed by skin biopsy, typically performed with local anesthesia using 1 of 3 techniques: saucerization shave biopsy, punch biopsy, or narrow excision with 2-mm margins. A narrow excision to the subdermal fat without undermining is preferred to avoid disruption of lymphatics because this can impair future sentinel lymph node biopsy (SLNB). On a limb, the scar should be oriented along the long axis. The biopsy should assess the invasion depth (Breslow thickness) because this is the most important prognostic indicator and guides treatment.[16] In general, biopsy of the entire lesion is ideal to avoid sampling error, although this may be impractical for certain locations or large lesions. Data suggest that although shave and punch biopsies more commonly transect tumors than excision, there is no adverse effect on survival.[17]

For patients with an unknown primary skin lesion presenting with a bulky lymph node or metastatic disease, fine-needle aspiration may be used with sensitivity and specificity above 90%.[18] There are rare reports of tumor seeding along the biopsy tract so it should be monitored clinically for recurrence.[18] If clinical suspicion is high and the fine-needle aspiration is nondiagnostic, an excisional biopsy should be performed to confirm the diagnosis.[18] Tissue confirmation is needed even in the setting of distant metastatic disease, and molecular sequencing for common mutations is now standard of care.

Histopathology of CM reveals increased atypical melanocytes/melanoma cells in the epidermis and/or dermis. Atypical melanocytes may be seen higher up in the epidermis, termed, *pagetoid spread*, and there also may be continuous atypical melanocytes along the dermal-epidermal junction, termed *lentiginous proliferation*.[19]

Markers for melanocytic differentiation may be used to highlight melanocytes, including HMB-45, Melan-A/Mart 1, MITF, and Sox-10. Diagnosis is not always clear-cut and the term, *melanocytic tumor of uncertain malignant potential*, is used for lesions difficult to distinguish from melanoma, such as Spitz tumors, cellular and/or epithelioid blue nevi, and deep penetrating nevi.[20] Such lesions should be excised completely given their uncertain malignant potential. The Melanocytic Pathology Assessment Tool and Hierarchy for Diagnosis reporting schema attempt to consolidate discordant terminology with coordinated treatment of melanocytic lesions based on biological potential.[21]

STAGING

The American Joint Committee on Cancer (AJCC) unveiled its eighth edition of melanoma staging to be implemented at the beginning of January 2018. The samples included in the eighth edition are stages I–III CM diagnosed since 1998.[22] Notably, stage IV patients were not updated in this edition in anticipation of changes in survival due to recent therapeutics. The strict requirement of a SLNB for all tumors T2 and above, and the inclusion of the nodal status if an SLNB was adhered to, resulted in an improved overall survival (OS) status for stage I and stage II patients because patients with occult nodal metastases were appropriately staged as stage III (**Table 1**). The staging system continues to include tumor depth, nodal status, and presence of metastases (TNM) (**Table 2**).

Changes in Tumor Staging

The major change in tumor staging is defining T1a as less than 0.8 mm and T1b as greater than 0.8 mm or less than 0.8 mm but ulcerated (previous transition point set at 1 mm in the seventh edition). Mitotic rate was removed because analyses revealed

Table 1
Survival percentages by TNM staging

American Joint Committee on Cancer, Eighth Edition	5-y Survival (%)	10-y Survival (%)
Stage IA	99	98
Stage IB	97	94
Stage IIA	94	88
Stage IIB	87	82
Stage IIC	82	75
Stage IIIA	93	88
Stage IIIB	83	77
Stage IIIC	69	60
Stage IIID	32	24
American Joint Committee on Cancer, Seventh Edition		**1-y Survival (%)**
Stage IV M1a		62
Stage M1b		53
Stage M1c		33

Data from Balch CM, Gershenwald JE, Soong SJ, et al. Final version of 2009 AJCC melanoma staging and classification. J Clin Oncol 2009;27(36):6199–206; and Gershenwald JE, Scolyer RA. Melanoma staging: American Joint Committee on Cancer (AJCC) 8th edition and beyond. Ann Surg Oncol 2018;25(8):2105–10.

Table 2
TNM staging, American Joint Committee on Cancer, eighth edition

Tumor Classification	Thickness (mm)	Ulceration Status
T1	≤1.0	T1a, <0.8 mm without ulceration T1b, 0.8 mm to 1 mm without ulceration Or ≤1.0 mm with ulceration
T2	1.1–2.0	T2a, without ulceration T2b, with ulceration
T3	2.1–4.0	T3a, without ulceration T3b, with ulceration
T4	>4.0	T4a, without ulceration T4b, with ulceration

Nodal Classification	Number of Nodes	Clinical Detectability/Microsatellite Metastases Status
N1	1	NX, regionnal nodes not accessed N0, no regional metastases detected N1a, clinically occult; no MSI N1b, clinically detected; no MSI N1c, 0 nodes; MSI present
N2	2–3	N2a, clinically occult; no MSI N2b, clinically detected; no MSI N2c, 1 node; MSI present
N3	>4	N3a, clinically occult; no MSI N3b, clinically detected or presence of any number of matted nodes; no MSI N3c, >2 nodes or any number of matted nodes; MSI present

Metastases Classification	Site	Serum Lactate Dehydrogenase
M1a–d	Skin/subcutaneous/nodule (M1a); lung (M1b); visceral (M1c); CNS (M1d)	Not assessed
M1a–d(0)	Skin/subcutaneous/nodule (M1a); lung (M1b); visceral (M1c); CNS (M1d)	Normal
M1a–d(1)	Skin/subcutaneous/nodule (M1a); lung (M1b); visceral (M1c); CNS (M1d)	Elevated

T0 = no known primary.
Tis = melanoma in situ.
(sn), add to nodal status if SLN positive but completion lymphadenectomy not performed.
Abbreviation: MSI, microsatellite, satellite, and in-transit metastases.
Data from Gershenwald JE, Scolyer RA. Melanoma staging: American Joint Committee on Cancer (AJCC) 8th edition and beyond. Ann Surg Oncol 2018;25(8):2105–10; and Gormally MV. New Haven (CT).

that 0.8-mm tumor thickness carried more prognostic significance than the presence or absence of a mitotic figure.[22] Nonetheless, mitotic rate should still be recorded, because over the entire range of mitoses, there is predictive value that will likely be further elucidated in future studies. The relevance of determining T1a/b status is the difference between less than 5% likelihood of SLN metastases versus 5% to 12%.[22] Therefore T1b is the cutoff at which SLNB is recommended (discussed later).

Changes in Nodal Staging

The major change in the staging of nodal status in melanoma is the inclusion of the tumor status in the overall staging. In the seventh edition, the presence of nodal status trumped whatever tumor stage was associated with it. The inclusion of tumor thickness and ulceration results in a more granular distribution of stage III staging, from 3 to 4 categories (stages IIIA, IIIB, IIIC, and IIID) (**Table 3**). Previous terms, *microscopic* and *macroscopic* metastases, are now termed, *clinically occult*, if the nodal metastases are detected by SLNB, versus *clinically evident*, if they are detected by clinical or radiographic examination. Finally, the presence of microsatellites, satellites, or in-transit metastases is automatically under N1c, N2c, and N3c depending on the number of tumor-involved lymph nodes (1, 2 or 3, and 4 or more respectively). Microsatellites are defined as microscopic cutaneous or subcutaneous tumors discontiguous from the primary but found on pathologic examination of the original primary site.

Changes in Metastases Staging

The major changes in the staging of metastases status in melanoma are (1) the addition of central nervous system (CNS) metastases as a new class, Md, and (2) the inclusion of LDH as an additional prognostic factor to each M stage.

Mutational Subtyping of Melanoma

Exomic sequencing of metastatic melanoma is regularly performed to determine key mutations that will influence treatment and prognosis. The Cancer Genome Atlas Network recently provided a schema for CM classification: *BRAF*, *RAS*, *NF-1*, and

Table 3
TNM staging, clinical stage American Joint Committee on Cancer, eighth edition, continued

Stage 0	Tis	N0	M0
Stage IA	T1a	N0	M0
Stage IB	T1b	N0	M0
	T2a	N0	M0
Stage IIA	T2b	N0	M0
	T3a	N0	M0
Stage IIB	T3b	N0	M0
	T4a	N0	M0
Stage IIC	T4b	N0	M0
Stage IIIA	T1a–T2a	N1a	M0
	T1a–T2a	N1b	M0
Stage IIIB	T0–T3a	N1b–N1c	M0
	T2b–T3a	N2a	M0
	T1a–T3a	N2b	M0
Stage IIIC	T3b–T4a	N1a–N2b	M0
	T0	N2b–N3c	M0
	Any T	N2c	M0
	T1a–T4a	N2c–N3c	M0
	T4b	N2c	M0
Stage IIID	T4b	N3a–N3c	M0
Stage IV	Any T	Any N	M1

Data from Gershenwald JE, Scolyer RA. Melanoma Staging: American Joint Committee on Cancer (AJCC) 8th Edition and Beyond. Ann Surg Oncol 2018;25(8):2105–10; and Gormally MV. New Haven (CT).

triple–wild type (WT)[23] (**Table 4**). Increasingly genomic classification will likely replace the current pathologic subtyping system of superficial spreading, nodular, acral-lentiginous, and LM melanomas. Mutational status of a patient's tumor represents a move toward personalized medicine both from prognostic and treatment points of view. The best example to date remains the highly selective targeting of the kinase domain of *BRAF* resulting in cessation of *BRAFV600* mutant metastatic melanoma.[24] In **Table 4**, treatment options specific to the listed mutations that have clinical relevance are provided, with many more that have demonstrated efficacy that are not included.

Molecular Predictors of Melanoma Outcome

The need for additional prognosticators beyond SLN is clear because further risk-stratifying early-stage tumors (stage I and II) currently is not possible. A recent study has highlighted the burden of mortality in stage I melanomas comprising 23% of all melanoma-related deaths in Queensland, Australia, even though the 10-year survival for stage I melanoma patients is 94% to 98%.[25] Circulating factors, cell-free DNA, tumor-infiltrating lymphocytes, and other immune biomarkers have all been investi-gated for prognostic ability in melanoma outcome. In addition, gene expression pro-files, such as what has been released by Castle Biosciences, Inc., (Phoenix, AZ), has been shown to be an independent predictor of metastatic risk, including in pa-tients with negative SLN biopsies.[26] This platform is available for clinical use, but as-sociation with improved patient survival or alteration in outcome as a result of the testing has not yet been demonstrated. Although there likely will be molecular predic-tors in the near future, none are currently recommended by major collective cancer groups, such as the NCCN or AJCC.

SURGICAL MANAGEMENT AND RADIATION

Initial definitive surgical management of CM with wide local excision (WLE) is critical to reduce local recurrence and melanoma-specific mortality. Recent data have

Table 4
Genomic classification of cutaneous melanoma

Gene	Hot Spot Mutations	Percentage	Characteristics	Treatment
BRAF	BRAFV600E, K	35–50	• Early driver mutation also seen in benign nevi (80%) • Younger patients	Combination BRAF and MEK inhibition
RAS	Q61K, Q61R	10–25	• Associated with thicker tumors, higher mitotic rate • Associated with nodular subtype	MEK inhibition
NF-1	—	14	• Older patients • High mutational burden	—
Triple WT	*c-KIT; GNAQ*	10	• Lack UV signature • Increased copy number alteration, structural rearrangements • Acral lentiginous, mucosal subtype	c-KIT inhibition

Data from Refs.[23,55,56]

suggested that mortality is improved when stage I patients undergo WLE within 30 days of initial biopsy, but no effect was seen for stage II and stage III patients.[27] The primary goal of WLE is tumor removal, with secondary goals of minimizing surgical site complications and cosmetic disfigurement.

Prior to the 1970s, WLE was empirically performed with margins up to 5 cm, but data from several RCTs suggest rates of local control and survival with narrower margins.[28] The recommended peripheral clinical margins for WLE depend on the Breslow thickness and range from 0.5 cm to 2.0 cm (**Table 5**).[29] The depth should be to the fascia; data suggest no additional benefit from deeper excision.[28] For LM, a type of melanoma in situ, the debate on the ideal surgical margin persists.

Breslow thickness predicts the likelihood of SLN metastases. The Multicenter Selective Lymphadenectomy Trial (MSLT) I examined SLNB in intermediate-thickness melanoma (1.2–3.5 mm) and found a positivity rate of 16.0%.[30] Additionally, SLN positivity was found the single most important prognostic factor.[30] For thin melanoma less than 1.0 mm, a depth greater than 0.75 mm is associated with a higher rate of SLNB positivity (6.2% vs 2.7%),[31] although the prognostic value is less clear.[29] Current guidelines recommend SLNB for melanoma staged T1b and greater (eg, < 0.8-mm thick with ulceration or ≥ 0.8-mm thick with or without ulceration).[29] The exception is pure desmoplastic melanoma, which tends to have lower rates of SLN positivity; thus, the role of SLNB in these cases is controversial.[29]

Historically, patients with a positive SLNB subsequently underwent complete lymph node dissection (CLND). This practice, however, has recently been challenged by the results of the MSLT II, which randomized patients with SLN positivity to CLND or observation with frequent nodal ultrasonography (every 4 months for 2 years then every 6 months for years 3–5) and CLND only if there was nodal recurrence.[32] The MSLT II found that immediate CLND increased the rate of regional control (92% vs 77%) and improved disease-free survival slightly (68% vs 63%), but melanoma-specific survival was unaffected (86% vs 86%).[32] Lymphedema was a significant complication in the group undergoing CLND (24.1% vs 6.3%).[32] Given CLND's morbidity and lack of survival benefit, the authors' institution forgoes immediate CLND and conducts active surveillance in patients with SLNB positivity using nodal ultrasonography as per the MSLT II timeframe.[32] Therapeutic lymphadenectomy is performed when there is nodal recurrence confirmed by FNA and no evidence of distant metastases, or if there is a bulky nodal disease.

For patients with resectable in-transit metastases without distant metastases, surgical excision is recommended to obtain pathologic clearance, but WLE margins are unnecessary.[29] For in-transit metastases not amenable to resection, treatment options include topical imiquimod, intralesional talimogene laherparepvec (T-VEC), and

Table 5	
Surgical margins for wide local excision of primary melanoma	
Breslow Thickness	**Peripheral Clinical Surgical Margins**
In situ	0.5–1.0 cm
<1.0 mm	1.0 cm
1.0–2.0 mm	1.0–2.0 cm
> 2.0 mm	2.0 cm

Adapted from Richard GBH, Langley. Skin cancer: an overview of non-melanoma cancers and melanoma. 3rd edition. Halifax (Canada); Cancer Care Nova Scotia: 2013; with permission.

radiation therapy (RT).[29] In patients with in-transit as well as distant metastatic disease, systemic treatment options should be considered.

RT is not typically used first line but is useful in select clinical scenarios. For unresectable LM, RT may be used with clearance rates reported of 83% when used in isolation and 90% when used in conjunction with partial surgical clearance.[33] Topical imiquimod also has high reported clearance rates clinically and histologically for unresectable LM (70% to 100%), although a phase 2 study demonstrated a complete clearance rate of 37% with imiquimod as a monotherapy in the treatment of LM.[29,34] RT may also be used in the adjuvant setting for primary melanomas where anatomic constraints prevent clear surgical margins (eg, head and neck). For desmoplastic melanoma, a locally aggressive subtype, RT may have an adjuvant role both for positive surgical margins and for negative surgical margins in the setting of high-risk features, such as neurotropism or Breslow thickness of 4 mm or greater.[35] Palliative RT also can be useful for metastases, in particular stereotactic radiosurgery or whole-brain radiation for brain metastases.

MEDICAL MANAGEMENT OF METASTATIC MELANOMA
Immunotherapy

In 2011, ipilimumab, a CTLA-4 inhibitor, was approved by the FDA for the treatment of metastatic melanoma, ushering in an era of therapeutics that reverse the immune system's natural ability to turn itself off. Prior to this, the last therapeutic approved for metastatic melanoma was interleukin 2 in 1998. CM is a known immunogenic tumor as evidence of regression is seen both clinically and pathologically. Previous attempts at immunotherapy and vaccination treatments focused on boosting immune response by increasing the number or efficacy of cytotoxic T cells. The recent wave of immunotherapy targets CTLA-4 and the programmed cell death protein 1(PD-1)/programmed death-ligand 1(PDL-1) pathways, immunomodulatory receptors expressed on T cells. These receptors and their ligands regulate T-cell exhaustion and the blockade of this pathway can revive exhausted CD8$^+$ cells. This normal compensatory pathway, important in chronic infections, is hijacked by tumor cells, such as those found in melanoma.

The initial phase III study demonstrated superiority of ipilimumab over glycoprotein (gp) 100 vaccine with an improved median OS (10 months vs 6.4 months).[36] Grade 3 or grade 4 immune-related events (IREs) were noted, however, in 10% to 15% of the ipilimumab arm (vs 3% in gp100 alone). Ipilimumab responders demonstrate a unique aspect of checkpoint blockade—responders frequently (20%) are long-term responders with the plateau starting at 3 years.[37] The PD-1 inhibitors, nivolumab and pembrolizumab, came shortly thereafter, and were demonstrated to have higher response rates as well as decreased incidence of grade 3 to grade 4 side effects. Nivolumab as a monotherapy in previously untreated *BRAF* WT patients compared with dacarbazine has a response rate of 40%, 1-year survival rate of 72.9% (vs 42.1), and a grade 3 or grade 4 adverse event rate of 11.7%.[38,39]

In a phase 3 study, the combination of nivolumab and ipilimumab proved superior to ipilimumab alone or nivolumab alone in terms of median progression-free survival (PFS) (11.5 months vs 2.9 months vs 6.9 months, respectively).[40,41] Combination therapy also had the highest response rate at 57.6% (compared with 43.7% nivolumab and 19% ipilimumab). At the 3-year update, the OS rate was 58% in the combination group and 52% in the nivolumab group compared with 34% in the ipilimumab group.[42] Treatment-related adverse events of grade 3 or grade 4 occurred in 59% of the patients in the combination group (vs 21% nivolumab and 28% ipilimumab). Taken together, the combination therapy offers a superior response rate but modestly better

OS compared with PD-1 inhibition alone with a higher IRE profile. As a result, not all patients receive combination therapy as first-line therapy.

The adverse event profile of immunotherapy is beyond the scope of this review, but the significance of having an IRE is important in that there are several lines of evidence suggesting a correlation between having an IRE and a disease response. For instance, in the 120 patients who discontinued combination therapy due to toxic effects, 67.5% had a response.[41] Predictors of response to immunotherapy is also an area of active investigation. Finally, several other checkpoint pathways are being studied in combination with CTLA-4 and PD-1 inhibition.

Targeted Therapy

The development of a highly selective oral inhibitor of BRAFV600E mutation was ground-breaking and heralded an influx of other highly specific kinase-targeting agents in all cancer treatment.[24] Although BRAF-inhibition (BRAFi) as a monotherapy for BRAFV600 mutant unresectable melanoma, was associated with a high response rate (approximately 50%) and a rapid onset (within 2 weeks), it was also almost universally associated with relapse with a median PFS of 6 months to 8 months.[43] This acquired resistance was due to paradoxical activation of the MAPK pathway. Combination therapy using both BRAFi and MEK-inhibition (MEKi) seems to negate the resistance pathways. In a phase 3 trial comparing dabrafenib/tramatenib to vemurafenib in previously untreated patients, combination therapy demonstrated improved OS of 72% versus 65% at 12 months.[44] The combination therapy also had improved response rate (64% vs 51%) and improved median PFS (11.4 months vs 7.3 months).[44] This study confirmed several other previous combination versus monotherapy studies that all concurred the superiority of combination therapy in the treatment of BRAFV600 mutant melanoma.[45,46] The current FDA-approved BRAFi/MEKi combinations include vemurafenib/cobimetinib; dabrafenib/tramatenib; and encorafenib/binimetinib.

The question of whether to start with targeted therapy versus immunotherapy is an important question that reflects clinical judgment and may be further teased out as more data on sequential treatments are analyzed. Of course, BRAF WT patients would not benefit from targeted therapy. Often, checkpoint blockade is used as first line given the high response rate and durable responses. In patients with BRAFV600E mutant melanoma and rapidly growing tumor, the kinetics of targeted therapy are much faster (in the order of weeks) compared with immunotherapy (months, and sometimes with a delayed effect), and often are used to provide symptomatic relief to a patient.

Additional targeted therapy treatments, such as the treatment of c-kit mutant melanomas with c-kit inhibitors like imatinib mesylate, are not discussed in this review.

Adjuvant Therapy

Demonstrated efficacy of these medications soon led to trials in the adjuvant setting.

In the adjuvant setting, pembrolizumab has demonstrated to be superior than ipilimumab and with a lower adverse event rate. A head-to-head phase III study of pembrolizumab (3 mg/kg weight every 2 weeks) versus ipilimumab (10 mg/kg every 3 weeks for 4 doses and then every 12 weeks) in the adjuvant setting was completed for patients undergoing complete resection of stage IIIB, stage IIIC, or stage IV disease.[47,48] At 12 months, recurrence-free survival was 70.5% in the nivolumab group and 60.8% in the ipilimumab group. Treatment-related grade 3 or grade 4 adverse events were lower in the nivolumab arm (14.4% vs 45.9%).

The combination BRAFi/MEKi, has also been approved for adjuvant treatment of BRAFV600E and V600K stage III patients after complete resection based on data from the phase III COMBI-AD study.[49] At 3-year follow-up, patients on the treatment arm had an improved relapse-free survival compared with placebo (58% vs 39%).

SURVEILLANCE AND PREVENTION

All CM patients should undergo at least annual dermatologic examination indefinitely.[29] Approximately 2% to 10% of patients develop a second primary CM, approximately half of which occur within 1 year.[29] In addition to the risk of additional CM, patients are at risk for local and distant recurrence, although there is no proven survival benefit from earlier detection of recurrence.[29] Compared with later-stage melanoma, earlier-stage melanoma is less likely to recur but does so over a longer time horizon.[29] Current guidelines recommend that patients with stage IA to stage IIA melanoma undergo history, physical, and skin examination every 6 to 12 months for 5 years and annually thereafter.[29] Patients with stage IIB–IV melanoma should undergo such examination every 3 to 12 months for 3 years and annually thereafter.[29] In these patients, surveillance CT chest, abdomen, pelvis or PET/CT in addition to brain MRI may also be considered for the first 3 years postdiagnosis.[29]

Sun protection plays a key role in primary prevention of CM. A randomized controlled trial found reduced CM incidence (hazard ratio 0.50) in subjects randomized to daily rather than discretionary sunscreen use.[50] Numerous agents have been proposed for primary chemoprevention, including topical retinoids, polypodium leucotomos extract, nonsteroidal anti-inflammatory agents, and statins, but evidence is lacking to support regular use.[51] A meta-analysis found no association between vitamin D intake via diet and/or supplementation and CM incidence.[52] Vitamin D deficiency, however, is associated with worse prognosis in metastatic melanoma,[53] and a clinical trial is under way to examine vitamin D supplementation for tertiary prevention.[54] Given recommended sun-avoidant behavior, the authors regularly recommend vitamin D supplementation in CM patients.

REFERENCES

1. Institute NC. SEER cancer stat facts: melanoma of the skin.
2. Australia C. Melanoma of the skin statistics.
3. Bleyer A, Viny A, Barr R. Epidemiology, access, and outcomes: SEER series cancer in 15- to 29-year-olds by primary site. Oncologist 2006;11:590–601.
4. Guy GPJ, Thomas CC, Thompson T, et al. Vital signs: melanoma incidence and mortality trends and projections - United States, 1982-2030. MMWR Morb Mortal Wkly Rep 2015;64(21):591–6.
5. Boniol M, Autier P, Boyle P, et al. Cutaneous melanoma attributable to sunbed use: systematic review and meta-analysis. BMJ 2012;345(2):e4757.
6. El Ghissassi F, Baan R, Straif K, et al. A review of human carcinogens–part D: radiation. Lancet Oncol 2009;10(8):751–2.
7. Cust AE, Harland M, Makalic E, et al. Melanoma risk for CDKN2A mutation carriers who are relatives of population-based case carriers in Australia and the UK. J Med Genet 2011;48(4):266–72.
8. Chang AE, Karnell LH, Menck HR. The national cancer data base report on cutaneous and noncutaneous melanoma. Cancer 1998;83(8):1664–78.
9. Aitken JF, Elwood M, Baade PD, et al. Clinical whole-body skin examination reduces the incidence of thick melanomas. Int J Cancer 2010;126(2):450–8.
10. Bibbins-Domingo K, Grossman DC, Curry SJ, et al. Screening for skin cancer. JAMA 2016;316(4):429.

11. Breitbart EW, Waldmann A, Nolte S, et al. Systematic skin cancer screening in Northern Germany. J Am Acad Dermatol 2012;66(2):201–11.
12. Herschorn A. Dermoscopy for melanoma detection in family practice. Can Fam Physician 2012;58(7):740–5, e372-8.
13. Vestergaard ME, Macaskill P, Holt PE, et al. Dermoscopy compared with naked eye examination for the diagnosis of primary melanoma: a meta-analysis of studies performed in a clinical setting. Br J Dermatol 2008;159(3):669–76.
14. Rademaker M, Oakley A. Digital monitoring by whole body photography and sequential digital dermoscopy detects thinner melanomas. J Prim Health Care 2010;2(4):268–72.
15. Cinotti E, Labeille B, Debarbieux S, et al. Dermoscopy vs. reflectance confocal microscopy for the diagnosis of lentigo maligna. J Eur Acad Dermatol Venereol 2018;32(8):1284–91.
16. Gershenwald JE, Scolyer RA, Hess KR, et al. Melanoma staging: evidence-based changes in the American joint committee on cancer eighth edition Cancer Staging Man. CA Cancer J Clin 2018;67(6):472–92.
17. Mir M, Chan CS, Khan F, et al. The rate of melanoma transection with various biopsy techniques and the influence of tumor transection on patient survival. J Am Acad Dermatol 2013;68(3):452–8.
18. Hall BJ, Schmidt RL, Sharma RR, et al. Fine-needle aspiration cytology for the diagnosis of metastatic melanoma: Systematic review and meta-analysis. Am J Clin Pathol 2013;140(5):635–42.
19. Elder DE. Pathology of melanoma. Surg Oncol Clin N Am 2015;24(2):229–37.
20. Cerroni L, Barnhill R, Elder D, et al. Melanocytic tumors of uncertain malignant potential: Results of a tutorial held at the XXIX symposium of the international society of dermatopathology in Graz, October 2008. Am J Surg Pathol 2010;34(3):314–26.
21. Piepkorn MW, Barnhill RL, Elder DE, et al. The MPATH-Dx reporting schema for melanocytic proliferations and melanoma. J Am Acad Dermatol 2014;70(1):131–41.
22. Gershenwald JE, Scolyer RA. Melanoma staging: American Joint Committee on Cancer (AJCC) 8th Edition and Beyond. Ann Surg Oncol 2018;25(8):2105–10.
23. Akbani R, Akdemir KC, Aksoy BA, et al. Genomic classification of cutaneous melanoma. Cell 2015;161(7):1681–96.
24. Flaherty KT, Puzanov I, Kim KB, et al. Inhibition of mutated, activated BRAF in metastatic melanoma. N Engl J Med 2009;361(2):809–19.
25. Whiteman DC, Baade PD, Olsen CM. More people die from thin melanomas (≤1 mm) than from thick melanomas (>4 mm) in Queensland, Australia. J Invest Dermatol 2015;135(4):1190–3.
26. Gastman BR, Gerami P, Kurley SJ, et al. Identification of patients at risk for metastasis using a prognostic 31-gene expression profile in subpopulations of melanoma patients with favorable outcomes by standard criteria. J Am Acad Dermatol 2018. [Epub ahead of print].
27. Conic RZ, Cabrera CI, Khorana AA, et al. Determination of the impact of melanoma surgical timing on survival using the National Cancer Database. J Am Acad Dermatol 2018;78(1):40–6.e7.
28. Testori A, Rutkowski P, Marsden J, et al. Surgery and radiotherapy in the treatment of cutaneous melanoma. Ann Oncol 2009;20(SUPPL. 4):22–9.
29. Fleming MD. NCCN evidence blocks TM. 2017:2016. doi:10.1007/978-1-84996-314-5.

30. Morton DL, Thompson JF, Cochran AJ, et al. Sentinel-node biopsy or nodal obser-vation in melanoma. N Engl J Med 2006;355(13):1307–17.
31. Andtbacka RHI, Gershenwald JE. Role of sentinel lymph node biopsy in patients with thin melanoma. J Natl Compr Cancer Netw 2009;7(3):308–17.
32. Faries MB, Thompson JF, Cochran AJ, et al. Completion dissection or observation for sentinel-node metastasis in melanoma. N Engl J Med 2017;376(23):2211–22.
33. Hedblad M-A, Mallbris L. Grenz ray treatment of lentigo maligna and early lentigo maligna melanoma. J Am Acad Dermatol 2012;67(1):60–8.
34. Marsden JR, Fox R, Boota NM, et al. Effect of topical imiquimod as primary treat-ment for lentigo maligna: the LIMIT-1 study. Br J Dermatol 2017;176(5):1148–54.
35. Oliver DE, Patel KR, Parker D, et al. The emerging role of radiotherapy for desmo-plastic melanoma and implications for future research. Melanoma Res 2015; 25(2):95–102.
36. Hodi FS, Sosman JA, Haanen JB, et al. Improved survival with ipilimumab in pa-tients with metastatic melanoma 2010;363(8):711–23.
37. Schadendorf D, Hodi FS, Robert C, et al. Pooled analysis of long-term survival data from phase II and phase III trials of ipilimumab in unresectable or metastatic melanoma. J Clin Oncol 2015;33(17):1889–94.
38. Robert C, Long GV, Brady B, et al. Nivolumab in previously untreated melanoma without BRAF mutation. N Engl J Med 2015;372(4):320–30.
39. Weber JS, D'Angelo SP, Minor D, et al. Nivolumab versus chemotherapy in pa-tients with advanced melanoma who progressed after anti-CTLA-4 treatment (CheckMate 037): a randomised, controlled, open-label, phase 3 trial. Lancet On-col 2015;16(4):375–84.
40. Postow MA, Chesney J, Pavlick AC, et al. Nivolumab and ipilimumab versus ipi-limumab in untreated melanoma. N Engl J Med 2015;372(21):2006–17.
41. Larkin J, Chiarion-Sileni V, Gonzalez R, et al. Combined nivolumab and ipilimu-mab or monotherapy in untreated melanoma. N Engl J Med 2015;373(1):23–34.
42. Wolchok JD, Chiarion-Sileni V, Gonzalez R, et al. Overall survival with combined nivolumab and ipilimumab in advanced melanoma. N Engl J Med 2017;377(14): 1345–56.
43. Chapman PB, Hauschild A, Robert C, et al. Improved survival with vemurafenib in melanoma with BRAF V600E mutation. N Engl J Med 2011;364(26):2507–16.
44. Robert C, Karaszewska B, Schachter J, et al. Improved overall survival in mela-noma with combined dabrafenib and trametinib. N Engl J Med 2015;372(1):30–9.
45. Larkin J, Ascierto PA, Dréno B, et al. Combined vemurafenib and cobimetinib in BRAF -mutated melanoma. N Engl J Med 2014;371(20):1867–76.
46. Long GV, Stroyakovskiy D, Gogas H, et al. Combined BRAF and MEK inhibition versus BRAF inhibition alone in melanoma. N Engl J Med 2014;371(20):1877–88.
47. Weber J, Mandala M, Del Vecchio M, et al. Adjuvant nivolumab versus ipilimumab in resected stage III or IV melanoma. N Engl J Med 2017. https://doi.org/10.1056/NEJMoa1709030.
48. Eggermont AMM, Blank CU, Mandala M, et al. Adjuvant pembrolizumab versus placebo in resected stage III melanoma. N Engl J Med 2018. https://doi.org/10.1056/NEJMoa1802357.
49. Long GV, Hauschild A, Santinami M, et al. Adjuvant dabrafenib plus trametinib in stage III BRAF -mutated melanoma. N Engl J Med 2017. https://doi.org/10.1056/NEJMoa1708539.
50. Green AC, Williams GM, Logan V, et al. Reduced melanoma after regular sun-screen use: Randomized trial follow-up. J Clin Oncol 2011;29(3):257–63.

51. Mounessa J, Buntinx-Krieg T, Qin R, et al. Primary and secondary chemoprevention of malignant melanoma. Am J Clin Dermatol 2016;17(6):625–34.
52. Caini S, Boniol M, Tosti G, et al. Vitamin D and melanoma and non-melanoma skin cancer risk and prognosis: a comprehensive review and meta-analysis. Eur J Cancer 2014;50(15):2649–58.
53. Timerman D, Mcenery-stonelake M, Joyce CJ, et al. Vitamin D deficiency is associated with a worse prognosis in metastatic melanoma 2017;8(4):6873–82.
54. De Smedt J, Van Kelst S, Boecxstaens V, et al. Vitamin D supplementation in cutaneous malignant melanoma outcome (ViDMe): a randomized controlled trial. BMC Cancer 2017;17(1):1–10.
55. Devitt B, Liu W, Salemi R, et al. Clinical outcome and pathological features associated with NRAS mutation in cutaneous melanoma. Pigment Cell Melanoma Res 2011;24(4):666–72.
56. Beadling C, Jacobson-Dunlop E, Hodi FS, et al. KIT gene mutations and copy number in melanoma subtypes. Clin Cancer Res 2008;14(21):6821–8.

Merkel Cell Carcinoma Review

Yun Xue, MD[a], Manisha Thakuria, MD[a,b],*

KEYWORDS

- Merkel cell carcinoma • Neuroendocrine tumor • Immunotherapy • Guidelines
- Merkel cell polyomavirus

KEY POINTS

- Merkel cell carcinoma (MCC) presents as rapidly growing tumors on sun-exposed areas, most commonly in elderly patients of light skin types and immunosuppressed patients.
- MCC tumors can be divided into virus-positive and virus-negative types, and patients with the former type can be monitored for recurrence using antibodies to viral antigens.
- MCC patients should receive interdisciplinary care, including surgical excision of the primary tumor, sentinel lymph node biopsy, adjuvant radiotherapy, and systemic therapy for metastatic disease.
- Checkpoint immunotherapy has become first-line standard of care for patients with advance-stage metastatic disease.
- The National Comprehensive Cancer Network provides the most up-to-date guidelines that should be used for the management of MCC patients.

INTRODUCTION

Merkel cell carcinoma (MCC) is a rare and aggressive cutaneous malignancy of neuroendocrine origin. It was first described in 1972 by Toker,[1] who named it "trabecular carcinoma of the skin" based on histopathologic patterns. It was a challenging and often missed diagnosis due to the wide histopathologic differential diagnosis of malignant small blue cell tumors. The advent of immunohistochemistry staining for cytokeratin (CK) 20, a shared neuroendocrine marker, greatly improved diagnostic accuracy. Over the past decade, staging, treatment, and surveillance of the cancer have progressed at a remarkably rapid pace. This article provides an update on the current guidelines around diagnosis and management and reviews the exciting advancements on the horizon.

Disclosure Statement: The authors declare that they have no conflicts of interest.
[a] Department of Dermatology, Brigham and Women's Hospital, Harvard Medical School, 221 Longwood Avenue, Boston, MA 02215, USA; [b] Department of Dermatology, Center for Cutaneous Oncology, Dana-Farber/Brigham and Women's Cancer Center, 450 Brookline Avenue, Boston, MA 02115, USA
* Corresponding author. 221 Longwood Avenue, Boston, MA 02215.
E-mail address: mthakuria1@bwh.harvard.edu

Hematol Oncol Clin N Am 33 (2019) 39–52
https://doi.org/10.1016/j.hoc.2018.08.002
0889-8588/19/© 2018 Elsevier Inc. All rights reserved.

PATHOGENESIS

Despite the growing body of research investigating the pathogenesis of MCC, the cell of origin is still under debate for this potentially mislabeled cancer. Tumor cells share morphologic and histologic features with the normal Merkel cell; however, Merkel cells are postmitotic and reside most densely in areas that are uncommon sites of MCC, such as palms and soles, oral and genital mucosa, and nail beds.[2] There is no evidence of direct evolution from normal Merkel cells into tumor cells and no described benign or dysplastic precursor lesions. Other proposed candidates for the cell of origin include a dermal or epidermal stem cell and a cell of B-cell lineage, but this remains an area of continued debate.[3]

In their landmark 2008 article, Feng and colleagues[4] described a novel polyomavirus, termed the Merkel cell polyomavirus (MCPyV), present in 8 of 10 MCC tumors and clonally integrated into the tumor genome in 6 of 8 tumors. This was the first association of a polyomavirus with human tumorigenesis. MCPyV is a double-stranded DNA virus in the *Polyomaviridae* family. It is ubiquitous in humans from a young age; 1 Italian study showed seropositivity for MCPyV in 41.7% of children ages 1 to 4 and 87.6% of young adults ages 15 to 19.[5]

The current model of pathogenesis divides MCCs into 2 types: virus positive and virus negative. Virus-positive tumors are found in 80% of cases in the northern hemisphere, whereas virus-negative tumors are found in a majority of southern hemisphere cases.[6] Tumor cells of these 2 categories have different mechanisms of promoting cell growth and replication.

In virus-positive tumors, MCPyV is integrated into the human genome, and viral oncoproteins named T-antigens are constitutively expressed to act on multiple pathways of cell growth, including inhibition of tumor-suppressor retinoblastoma protein, stabilization of oncoprotein c-Myc, and evasion of innate immunity.[7–10] Whole-transcriptome and genome sequencing of tumors has shown that viral integration sites overlap with focal genome amplifications, suggesting that despite a low mutation burden, the virus takes over the innate cell division mechanism to drive tumorigenesis.[11]

Virus-negative tumors, in contrast, accumulate a large number of somatic mutations via UV exposure.[12–14] Many of the mutations identified involved C > T and CC > TT substitutions, which are characteristic UV signatures also found in other cutaneous malignancies.[15] These mutations affect the tumor suppressor *p53* and *RB1* pathways as well as epigenetic factors that activate oncogenes.[13] Analysis of whole transcriptomes and genomes of primary MCC tumors reveals that all of these cumulative mutations lead to tumorigenesis in a very different pathway from viral-driven tumorigenesis, but the end result converges in a histologically indistinguishable tumor.[11]

EPIDEMIOLOGY

MCC disproportionately affects elderly individuals with a history of significant sun exposure and immunosuppression. Several population studies have shown that MCC occurs 62% of the time in men and 38% of the time in women[16–18]; 95% of all affected patients have light skin and more than 75% are older than age 65.[18,19] The incidence increases exponentially, ranging from 0.1 (per 100,000 person-years) in individuals ages 40 to 44, to 1.0 in those ages 60 to 64, and to 9.8 in those older than age 85.[16]

Immunosuppressed individuals tend to have a much higher risk of developing MCC even at younger ages. Solid organ transplant, for example, increases the risk of developing MCC by 24-fold.[20] This risk remains elevated over many decades due to the steady need for immunosuppressive medications. Individuals with HIV, chronic inflammatory disorders, or active malignancy are also at elevated risk compared with a cohort of comparable age.[21,22]

Since 2000, the overall incidence of MCC in the United States has increased by 95%, largely attributed to an aging population with weakened immune systems and more accurate diagnosis with CK20 staining in the 1990s.[16] In comparison, the incidence rates of melanoma and of all other solid tumors have risen by 57% and 15%, respectively. In 2013, the most recent estimated annual incidence rate was 0.7 cases per 100,000 people. It is projected that this incidence rate will continue to increase as the baby boomer generation ages.[16]

CLINICAL PRESENTATION

MCC typically presents as a rapidly growing, solitary, asymptomatic lesion. Crusting and ulceration are rarely found in early lesions. Although many are red-violet, firm, dome-shaped nodules located in sun-exposed areas, such as the head, neck, and extremities, they can be pleomorphic, appearing plaque-like, or as subcutaneous, flesh-colored nodules (**Fig. 1**). Their frequently innocuous appearance periodically results in misdiagnoses as cysts, lipomas, or other benign cutaneous lesions. In 2007, Heath and colleagues[17] found that 60 of 106 patients in their cohort had clinically benign-appearing lesions that were later confirmed to be MCC histologically. A majority of these lesions demonstrate 3 or more of the AEIOU features: asymptomatic nodule, expanding rapidly, in an immunosuppressed host, older than age 50, on UV-exposed sites or fair skin.[17]

At presentation, 65% of patients have skin-limited disease, 26% have nodal involvement, and 8% have distant metastases.[23] Spontaneous regression of the primary has occasionally been seen on re-excision specimens with a dense lymphocytic infiltrate of T cells around the site of the prior biopsy.[24] The most common sites of metastases are regional nodal basins, distant skin, lung, bone, and brain. There is a group of patients who present with nodal disease without an identifiable primary, with cases reported sporadically over the years.[25–27] Estimates show that approximately 40% of patients with clinically detectable nodal disease present without a known cutaneous primary, or approximately 4% of all cases of MCC.[23,28] The disease can present in

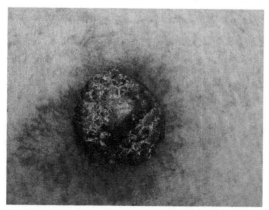

Fig. 1. Primary MCC presenting as scaly, papillomatous pink nodule on a pink patch of telangiectasias.

the inguinal, axillary, or head and neck nodes. Common sites of metastatic progression for these patients are similar to those with a known primary.[25]

One recent population study of 8765 cases showed that advanced stage at the time of diagnosis was associated with darker skin type, lack of medical insurance, residing far away from treatment facility, primary tumor located on the trunk or lower extremities, and undifferentiated tumor histology.[29] Patients who match these demographics may benefit from aggressive work-up and treatment to ensure optimal outcomes.

STAGING

Before 2009, there was a lack of consensus around staging and prognosis for MCC because the diagnosis was so rare and data regarding presentation, management, and outcomes were available from only a small number of patients. Different institutions developed their own tissue-node-metastasis staging systems with varied cutoff points, making it difficult for consensus classification and evaluation of outcomes based on initial presentation.

In 2009, the first ever American Joint Committee on Cancer (AJCC) consensus staging system for MCC was developed from the analysis of 5823 cases in the National Cancer Database (NCDB).[30] Stage I and stage II patients had skin-limited disease and were separated by size of primary tumor with the cutoff at 2 cm. Nodal disease was evaluated both clinically and pathologically. Patients were automatically upstaged if there was no pathologic evaluation of the node, such as with sentinel lymph node biopsy (SLNB) or completion lymph node dissection (eg, stage IA for patients with a small primary and a negative SLNB vs stage IB for patients with the same size primary but without pathologic evaluation of nodal tissue). Stage III patients included all with nodal disease and in-transit disease and were further subdivided by presence of microscopic nodal disease (stage IIIA) or macroscopic nodal disease (stage IIIB). Patients with in transit metastases were also included in stage IIIB. Stage IV patients had distant metastases.

In 2017, an analysis of 9387 patients with MCC diagnosed between 1998 and 2012 from the NCDB resulted in the revised AJCC staging system, 8th edition.[23] The updated system separates clinical and pathologic staging. The latter involves histologic examination of tissue, which results in more specific staging with implications for more accurate prognosis. Additionally, patients with nodal disease and an unknown primary were moved to a separate stage from node-positive patients with a known primary, because the former tends to have better prognosis.[28] The specific stages are summarized in **Table 1**.

Consideration of SLNB is indicated in all patients with clinically node-negative MCC because it allows for maximally guided management of regional disease. The impact of SLNB on survival has been mixed in the literature: patients with a negative SLNB had an 84.5% to 86.8% 5-year MCC-specific survival rate compared with 64.6% to 82.4% of patients with positive nodes.[31,32] The wide range of survival rates across studies of patients with positive SLNBs may reflect the variable institutional differences in management of regional disease. The rate of in-transit recurrences tend also to be higher in patients with a positive SLNB.[32] Approximately one-third of patients without clinical nodal involvement have microscopic involvement detected by SLNB.[30] One study, however, showed a false-negative rate of up to 17%, and regional recurrences have been seen in patients with negative SLNBs.[33] It is, therefore, important for SLNB to be performed at the time of local wide excision to ensure accurate identification of the draining nodal basin and for adjuvant radiation to still be considered for patients with negative SLNBs but high-risk primary tumors.

Table 1
American Joint Committee on Cancer, 8th edition, Merkel cell carcinoma staging system

Stage		Primary Tumor	Lymph Node	Metastasis
0		Tis: in situ (within epidermis only)	N0: no regional lymph node metastasis	M0: no distant metastasis
I	Clinical	T1: ≤2 cm maximum tumor dimension	N0: nodes negative by clinical examination (no pathologic examination performed)	M0: no distant metastasis
I	Pathologic	T1: ≤2 cm maximum tumor dimension	N0: nodes negative by pathologic examination	M0: no distant metastasis
IIA	Clinical	T2-3: >2 cm tumor dimension	N0: nodes negative by clinical examination (no pathologic examination performed)	M0: no distant metastasis
IIA	Pathologic	T2-3: >2 cm tumor dimension	N0: nodes negative by pathologic examination	M0: no distant metastasis
IIB	Clinical	T4: primary tumor invades bone, muscle, fascia, or cartilage	N0: nodes negative by clinical examination (no pathologic examination performed)	M0: no distant metastasis
IIB	Pathologic	T4: primary tumor invades bone, muscle, fascia, or cartilage	N0: nodes negative by pathologic examination	M0: no distant metastasis
III	Clinical	T0-4: any size/depth tumor	N1-3: nodes positive by clinical examination (no pathologic exam performed)	M0: no distant metastasis

(continued on next page)

Table 1
(continued)

Stage		Primary Tumor	Lymph Node	Metastasis
IIIA	Pathologic	T1–4: any size/depth tumor	N1a(sn) or N1a: nodes positive by pathologic examination only (nodal disease not apparent on clinical examination)	M0: no distant metastasis
		T0: not detected ("unknown primary")	N1b: nodes positive by clinical examination and confirmed via pathologic examination	M0: no distant metastasis
IIIB	Pathologic	T1–4: any size/depth tumor	N1b-3: nodes positive by clinical examination, and confirmed via pathologic examination OR in-transit metastasis	M0: no distant metastasis
IV	Clinical	T0–4: any	Any N: ±regional nodal involvement	M1: distant metastasis detected via clinical examination
IV	Pathologic	T0–4: any	Any N: ±regional nodal involvement	M1: distant metastasis confirmed via pathologic examination

Adapted from Harms KL, Healy MA, Nghiem P, et al. Analysis of prognostic factors from 9387 Merkel cell carcinoma cases forms the basis for the new 8th edition AJCC staging system. Ann Surg Oncol 2016;23(11):3564–71; with permission.

The practice of imaging for occult nodal and metastatic disease at the time of initial staging varies by institution. The current guidelines state that imaging studies should be performed when nodal disease is detected or as clinically indicated at the time of presentation. Although practices vary between institutions, contrast brain MRI plus contrast CT neck/chest/abdomen/pelvis or whole-body PET/CT is standard.[34] The authors' institution favors using PET/CT to identify and quantify macrometastatic nodal or distant disease. A systematic review and meta-analysis of 10 imaging studies showed that PET/CT had a sensitivity of 90% and specificity of 98% with an area under the receiver operating characteristic curve of 0.96 and no significant statistical heterogeneity.[35] Multiple studies have noted that positive findings on initial staging scans resulted in upstaging 16% to 26% of the time.[36–38] The most recent prospective study showed that treatment decisions were affected in 27.6% of cases, often due to occult primary, gross residual disease at the primary site, and subclinical nodal involvement.[28] All of this suggests that PET/CT may be preferred for routine staging work-up.

TREATMENT

The rarity of MCC has made prospective studies of treatment difficult. Historically, there has been a lack of consensus around the most effective treatment algorithm. It was not until 2009 that the National Comprehensive Cancer Network (NCCN) released guidelines, although practices around surgery, radiation, and systemic therapy continue to vary by institution.[39] The most recent NCCN guidelines recommend treatment algorithms based on whether the patient has clinically local, nodal, or metastatic disease at presentation.[40]

Patients with primary lesions generally undergo wide location excision with SLNB. Surgical margins are typically 1 cm to 2 cm, with significant consideration given to minimizing the time needed for wound healing before adjuvant radiation can be pursued. In patients with negative SLNBs, if the primary tumor is less than 1 cm, widely excised with negative resection margins, and contains no high-risk features, data suggest that no adjuvant therapy is needed. This was demonstrated in a single-institution analysis of 105 patients with primary tumors less than 2 cm in diameter, treated with surgery alone without adjuvant radiation, which resulted in a low 6% rate of local and satellite recurrence over 48 months.[41]

After surgical excision, patients with high-risk tumors should undergo 50 Gy to 66 Gy of adjuvant radiation to the primary site. High-risk features include greater than 1 cm, positive or insufficient surgical margins, lymphovascular invasion, location on the head and neck, and an immunocompromised patient.[42,43] Location in the head and neck region, where anatomic variation occurs frequently, can result in higher false-negative SLNB rates. Adjuvant radiation typically reduces local recurrence in these cases by treating microscopic disease, resulting in decreased local recurrence rate and reduced recurrences in local nodal basins.[43] In general, however, studies around the practice are retrospective in nature, and although several investigators have suggested improved locoregional control and survival rates with postoperative radiation, a systemic review in 2013 failed to generate a consensus on overall benefit.[44]

Management of patients with positive SLNBs usually starts with full-body imaging, if not already performed. The patient should be referred to a multidisciplinary tumor board for consultation regarding next steps in management, including discussion of nodal dissection versus radiation therapy to the nodal basin, and consideration of clinical trials.[34]

Patients who present with clinically positive nodes typically undergo fine-needle aspiration or core biopsy of the node for confirmation. Practices around treating gross nodal disease have varied from radiation only to selective lymphadenectomy followed by radiation to complete nodal basin dissections. Although there is no consensus, 1 cohort study of 24 patients in 2010 suggested that radiation alone had comparable 2-year regional recurrence-free survival rates to complete nodal dissection and radiation.[45] Although limited in power and lack of randomization, this study suggests that radiation alone may offer comparable efficacy with a more favorable side-effect profile compared with surgery for both microscopic and gross nodal disease.

Patients with distant metastatic disease should be referred expediently to a multidisciplinary tumor board. They may benefit from a combination of surgical excision for local debulking, radiation for palliation of symptoms or nodal disease, and/or systemic therapy, often through clinical trials. Historically, chemotherapy regimens were based on small cell lung cancer protocols, with carboplatin/cisplatin-etoposide the first-line agents. Treatment failure was followed by off-label use of anthracyclines, cyclophosphamide, vincristine, bleomycin, and 5-fluorouracil in various combinations. Although MCC is chemosensitive, responses tend not to be durable: median progression-free survival was only approximately 3 months.[46]

In more recent years, advancements in immunotherapy have greatly extended survival for patients with metastatic disease, particularly with the use of checkpoint immunotherapy involving the PD-1 (programmed death) and PD-L1 (programmed death-ligand) pathways. These agents are now the standard, first-line agents for metastatic MCC.

Avelumab, a monoclonal antibody to PD-L1, was approved by the Food and Drug Administration in March of 2017 and is the first systemic therapy specifically for use in metastatic MCC. The international multicenter phase II JAVELIN Merkel 200 trial showed a 32% overall response rate and 11% complete response rate in patients who had received and failed prior chemotherapy.[47] After 1 year of follow-up, 72% of responders continued to have progression-free survival.[48]

Pembrolizumab and nivolumab are both currently in phase II trials with promising results. In a study of 25 systemic therapy-naive patients, pembrolizumab induced 4 complete responses and 10 partial responses.[49] The objective response rate was 56%. At 33 weeks, only 2 of the 14 responding patients had relapsed. The largest study of nivolumab to date consisted of a mix of 25 systemic therapy-naive and previously treated patients[50]; 22 patients responded, with a higher percentage occurring in treatment-naive patients. Analysis of progression-free survival is ongoing.

In these studies, response was seen in both virus-positive and virus-negative tumors, although studies have suggested that PD-L1 expression is higher on virus-positive tumors.[12] Despite the success of immune therapy, there is a subset of patients who fail to respond. Approximately only 50% of virus-positive MCCs express PD-1 on tumor-infiltrating lymphocytes and PD-L1 on tumor cells, which may explain this phenomenon.[51] In the pembrolizumab study, however, response did not seem to correlate with PD-L1 expression. Current research areas of great interest include whether response to immune therapy can be induced and markers that predict treatment response.

Significant interest has also been generated around local delivery of immunotherapy via talimogene laherparepvec (TVEC), which is the first oncolytic viral immunotherapy approved by the Food and Drug Administration in 2015 for melanoma. TVEC is a genetically altered herpes simplex type I virus that selectively replicates in tumor cells and express human granulocyte-macrophage colony-stimulating factor, which activates dendritic cells to present tumor antigens and encourage an innate cell-mediated host response. There have been a few reported cases regarding the success of TVEC in treating advanced locoregional MCC in elderly patients who were not good surgical or chemotherapy candidates.[52] Primary nodules regressed and did not recur for 7 months to 11 months after the last dose. A multicenter phase II trial is under way to further investigate its success in treating MCC and other cutaneous tumors (NCT02819843).

Finally, targeted therapies remain an area of research for virus-negative MCC tumors dominated by mutations that are oncogenic. Several different pathways have been identified to in many virus-negative tumors as potential targets of therapy. Various case reports have detailed patient responses to medications targeting these pathways, but no large systemic trials have been conducted thus far. For the most part, different tumors may display different mutation profiles, and each patient may benefit from tumor sequencing to identify a personalized set of best targeted therapies.

PI3K/AKT-activating mutations have commonly been found in virus-negative tumors, and 1 case reported complete response to idelalisib in a stage IV MCC patient.[53,54] MLN0128 is a target of the mTOR pathway currently in phase II trial for advanced MCC (NCT02514824). Multikinase inhibitors are a third class of therapies with varied results. Pazopanib was reported to induce partial remission in a case report.[55] Cabozantinib was poorly tolerated and did not show any benefit, resulting in early cessation of the trial.[56] Imatinib has been studied in the past but failed to show any benefit, although there has been 1 case reported of clinical remission after treatment.[57,58]

SURVEILLANCE

MCC recurs most often within the first 2 years after diagnosis. NCCN guidelines suggest that patients should be monitored closely every 3 months to 6 months with full skin examinations and lymph node surveillance for the first 2 years, followed by every 6 months to 12 months afterward.[39] Routine imaging is recommended for patients at high-risk for recurrence and metastases. PET/CT may be preferable because metastases to the bone and bone marrow are particularly important to identify and can be missed on CT.[36]

The frequency of routine imaging is not standard, and the high costs and radiation exposures are less than ideal. One of the most exciting advances in surveillance is the discovery that antibodies produced against viral oncoproteins may be a marker of tumor activity and can potentially be used in conjunction with less frequent imaging for disease surveillance.

In 2010, Galloway and colleagues[59] found that antibodies recognizing MCPyV large and small tumor-associated antigens were present in 40.5% of patients with active disease and only 0.9% of a control population. In patients who had high titers, treatment success correlated with a rapid fall in titers whereas recurrent disease correlated with a rapid rise. More importantly, the rise of titers preceded clinical and imaging evidence of metastatic disease in certain patients, suggesting that these antibodies can be early markers of disease progression.[59]

A recent prospective study evaluated the predictive performance of these titers and found that falling titers had a negative predictive value of 97% and rising titers had a positive predictive value of 83%.[60] Seropositivity at time of diagnosis was also correlated to decreased risk of recurrence, independent of age, gender, stage at diagnosis, and immunosuppression. Because of these 2 studies, the NCCN guidelines now suggest measurement of baseline MCPyV oncoprotein antibodies as part of the initial work-up for its prognostic value post-treatment.[40]

PROGNOSIS

The most recent population study of 9387 MCC cases from the NCDB Participant User File showed that disease extent at time of presentation was predictive of 5-year overall survival rates: 51% (local disease), 35% (nodal disease), and 14% (distant disease).[23] Patients who are immunosuppressed, for example, those with active hematologic malignancy or need for immunosuppressive drugs, also tend to have poorer prognoses.[61,62]

The 2010 NCDB study of 5371 patients showed that the median survival rate of patients with unknown primaries and nodal disease was approximately 3.5 years, whereas the median survival rate of patients with known primaries and nodal disease was approximately 2 years.[30] Better prognosis in MCC patients with unknown primaries is attributed to a robust cell-mediated immune system in its ability to respond to the primary tumor.

On a more granular level, histologic reviews of primary MCC tumors have shown that low depth of tumor invasion, absence of lymphovascular invasion, and nodular tumor growth pattern are independently associated with better prognosis.[63,64] Several studies have explored whether expression of p63, a multifunctional transcription factor necessary for normal epithelial development that has been a prognostic marker in other cancers, may be helpful in MCC. Although the trend seems to suggest overall decreased survival, the magnitude is variable.[65,66]

Intratumor lymphocyte infiltration, in particular of the CD8+ type, has also been correlated with improved survival, which speaks to the important role of the host cell-mediated immunity in treating MCC.[67,68] Although this is true in both virus-positive and virus-positive tumors, virus positive tumors tend to have more lymphocyte infiltration, which is believed one of the primary reasons why patients with virus-positive tumors tend to respond better to immunotherapy and have better prognosis.

REFERENCES

1. Toker C. Trabecular carcinoma of the skin. Arch Dermatol 1972;105(1):107–10.
2. Moll I, Zieger W, Schmelz M. Proliferative Merkel cells were not detected in human skin. Arch Dermatol Res 1996;288(4):184–7. Available at: http://www.ncbi.nlm.nih.gov/pubmed/8967790. Accessed July 8, 2018.
3. Zur Hausen A, Rennspiess D, Winnepenninckx V, et al. Early B-cell differentiation in Merkel cell carcinomas: clues to cellular ancestry. Cancer Res 2013;73(16):4982–7.
4. Feng H, Shuda M, Chang Y, et al. Clonal integration of a polyomavirus in human merkel cell carcinoma. Science 2008;319(5866):1096–100.
5. Nicol JTJ, Robinot R, Carpentier A, et al. Age-specific seroprevalences of merkel cell polyomavirus, human polyomaviruses 6, 7, and 9, and trichodysplasia spinulosa-associated polyomavirus. Clin Vaccine Immunol 2013;20(3):363–8.
6. Paik JY, Hall G, Clarkson A, et al. Immunohistochemistry for Merkel cell polyomavirus is highly specific but not sensitive for the diagnosis of Merkel cell carcinoma in the Australian population. Hum Pathol 2011. https://doi.org/10.1016/j.humpath.2010.12.013.
7. Houben R, Shuda M, Weinkam R, et al. Merkel cell polyomavirus-infected Merkel cell carcinoma cells require expression of viral T antigens. J Virol 2010;84(14):7064–72.
8. Shuda M, Kwun HJ, Feng H, et al. Human Merkel cell polyomavirus small T antigen is an oncoprotein targeting the 4E-BP1 translation regulator. J Clin Invest 2011;121(9):3623–34.

9. Shahzad N, Shuda M, Gheit T, et al. The T antigen locus of Merkel cell polyoma-virus downregulates human Toll-like receptor 9 expression. J Virol 2013;87(23):13009–19.
10. Griffiths DA, Abdul-Sada H, Knight LM, et al. Merkel cell polyomavirus small T an-tigen targets the NEMO adaptor protein to disrupt inflammatory signaling. J Virol 2013;87(24):13853–67.
11. Starrett GJ, Marcelus C, Cantalupo PG, et al. Merkel cell polyomavirus exhibits dominant control of the tumor genome and transcriptome in virus-associated merkel cell carcinoma. MBio 2017. https://doi.org/10.1128/mBio.02079-16.
12. Wong SQ, Waldeck K, Vergara IA, et al. UV-associated mutations underlie the eti-ology of MCV-negative Merkel cell carcinomas. Cancer Res 2015. https://doi.org/10.1158/0008-5472.CAN-15-1877.
13. Harms PW, Vats P, Verhaegen ME, et al. The distinctive mutational spectra of polyomavirus-negative Merkel cell carcinoma. Cancer Res 2015. https://doi.org/10.1158/0008-5472.CAN-15-0702.
14. Goh G, Walradt T, Markarov V, et al. Mutational landscape of MCPyV-positive and MCPyV-negative Merkel cell carcinomas with implications for immunotherapy. Oncotarget 2016. https://doi.org/10.18632/oncotarget.6494.
15. Popp S, Waltering S, Herbst C, et al. UV-B-type mutations and chromosomal im-balances indicate common pathways for the development of Merkel and skin squamous cell carcinomas. Int J Cancer 2002. https://doi.org/10.1002/ijc.10321.
16. Paulson KG, Park SY, Vandeven NA, et al. Merkel cell carcinoma: Current US inci-dence and projected increases based on changing demographics. J Am Acad Dermatol 2018;78(3):457–63.e2.
17. Heath M, Jaimes N, Lemos B, et al. Clinical characteristics of Merkel cell carci-noma at diagnosis in 195 patients: the AEIOU features. J Am Acad Dermatol 2008;58(3):375–81.
18. Agelli M, Clegg LX. Epidemiology of primary Merkel cell carcinoma in the United States. J Am Acad Dermatol 2003. https://doi.org/10.1016/S0190-9622(03)02108-X.
19. Albores-Saavedra J, Batich K, Chable-Montero F, et al. Merkel cell carcinoma de-mographics, morphology, and survival based on 3870 cases: a population based study. J Cutan Pathol 2010. https://doi.org/10.1111/j.1600-0560.2009.01370.x.
20. Clarke CA, Robbins HA, Tatalovich Z, et al. Risk of Merkel cell carcinoma after solid organ transplantation. J Natl Cancer Inst 2015. https://doi.org/10.1093/jnci/dju382.
21. Kaae J, Hansen AV, Biggar RJ, et al. Merkel cell carcinoma: Incidence, mortality, and risk of other cancers. J Natl Cancer Inst 2010. https://doi.org/10.1093/jnci/djq120.
22. Engels EA, Frisch M, Goedert JJ, et al. Merkel cell carcinoma and HIV infection. Lancet 2002. https://doi.org/10.1016/S0140-6736(02)07668-7.
23. Harms KL, Healy MA, Nghiem P, et al. Analysis of prognostic factors from 9387 Merkel cell carcinoma cases forms the basis for the new 8th edition AJCC staging system. Ann Surg Oncol 2016;23(11):3564–71.
24. Vesely MJJ, Murray DJ, Neligan PC, et al. Complete spontaneous regression in Merkel cell carcinoma. J Plast Reconstr Aesthet Surg 2008. https://doi.org/10.1016/j.bjps.2006.10.020.
25. Tarantola TI, Vallow LA, Halyard MY, et al. Unknown primary Merkel cell carci-noma: 23 new cases and a review. J Am Acad Dermatol 2013;68(3):433–40.
26. Deneve JL, Messina JL, Marzban SS, et al. Merkel cell carcinoma of unknown pri-mary origin. Ann Surg Oncol 2012;19(7):2360–6.

27. Straka JA, Straka MB. A review of Merkel cell carcinoma with emphasis on lymph node disease in the absence of a primary site. Am J Otolaryngol 1997;18(1): 55–65. Available at: http://www.ncbi.nlm.nih.gov/pubmed/9006679. Accessed June 29, 2018.

28. Foote M, Veness M, Zarate D, et al. Merkel cell carcinoma: the prognostic implications of an occult primary in stage IIIB (nodal) disease. J Am Acad Dermatol 2012. https://doi.org/10.1016/j.jaad.2011.09.009.

29. Trofymenko O, Zeitouni NC, Kurtzman DJ. Factors associated with advanced stage merkel cell carcinoma at initial diagnosis and the use of radiation therapy: results from the national cancer database. J Am Acad Dermatol 2018. https://doi.org/10.1016/j.jaad.2018.03.019.

30. Lemos BD, Storer BE, Iyer JG, et al. Pathologic nodal evaluation improves prognostic accuracy in Merkel cell carcinoma: analysis of 5823 cases as the basis of the first consensus staging system. J Am Acad Dermatol 2010. https://doi.org/10.1016/j.jaad.2010.02.056.

31. Kachare SD, Wong JH, Vohra NA, et al. Sentinel lymph node biopsy is associated with improved survival in Merkel cell carcinoma. Ann Surg Oncol 2014;21(5): 1624–30.

32. Sims JR, Grotz TE, Pockaj BA, et al. Sentinel lymph node biopsy in Merkel cell carcinoma: The Mayo Clinic experience of 150 patients. Surg Oncol 2018; 27(1):11–7.

33. Gunaratne DA, Howle JR, Veness MJ. Sentinel lymph node biopsy in Merkel cell carcinoma: a 15-year institutional experience and statistical analysis of 721 reported cases. Br J Dermatol 2016. https://doi.org/10.1111/bjd.14240.

34. Anita Engh N, Hoffmann KG, Fisher K, et al. NCCN guidelines for Merkel cell carcinoma. 2018. Available at: https://www.nccn.org/professionals/physician_gls/pdf/mcc.pdf. Accessed June 29, 2018.

35. Treglia G, Dabbagh Kakhki VR, Giovanella L, et al. Diagnostic performance of fluorine-18-fluorodeoxyglucose positron emission tomography in patients with Merkel cell carcinoma: a systematic review and meta-analysis. Am J Clin Dermatol 2013. https://doi.org/10.1007/s40257-013-0040-x.

36. Hawryluk EB, O'Regan KN, Sheehy N, et al. Positron emission tomography/computed tomography imaging in Merkel cell carcinoma: a study of 270 scans in 97 patients at the Dana-Farber/Brigham and Women's Cancer Center. J Am Acad Dermatol 2013. https://doi.org/10.1016/j.jaad.2012.08.042.

37. Siva S, Byrne K, Seel M, et al. 18F-FDG PET provides high-impact and powerful prognostic stratification in the staging of Merkel cell carcinoma: a 15-year institutional experience. J Nucl Med 2013. https://doi.org/10.2967/jnumed.112.116814.

38. Poulsen M, Macfarlane D, Veness M, et al. Prospective analysis of the utility of 18-FDG PET in Merkel cell carcinoma of the skin: A Trans Tasman Radiation Oncology Group Study, TROG 09:03. J Med Imaging Radiat Oncol 2018;62(3): 412–9.

39. Miller SJ, Alam M, Andersen J, et al. Merkel cell carcinoma. J Natl Compr Canc Netw 2009;7(3):322–32.

40. Bichakjian CK, Olencki T, Aasi SZ, et al. Merkel cell carcinoma, version 1.2018, NCCN clinical practice guidelines in oncology. J Natl Compr Cancer Netw 2018;16(6):742–74.

41. Frohm ML, Griffith KA, Harms KL, et al. Recurrence and survival in patients with Merkel cell carcinoma undergoing surgery without adjuvant radiation therapy to the primary site. JAMA Dermatol 2016;152(9):1001.

42. Miller NJ, Bhatia S, Parvathaneni U, et al. Emerging and mechanism-based therapies for recurrent or metastatic Merkel cell carcinoma. Curr Treat Options Oncol 2013. https://doi.org/10.1007/s11864-013-0225-9.
43. Harrington C, Kwan W. Radiotherapy and conservative surgery in the locoregional management of merkel cell carcinoma: the British Columbia cancer agency experience. Ann Surg Oncol 2016. https://doi.org/10.1245/s10434-015-4812-9.
44. Hasan S, Liu L, Triplet J, et al. The role of postoperative radiation and chemoradiation in Merkel cell carcinoma: a systematic review of the literature. Front Oncol 2013. https://doi.org/10.3389/fonc.2013.00276.
45. Fang LC, Lemos B, Douglas J, et al. Radiation monotherapy as regional treatment for lymph node-positive merkel cell carcinoma. Cancer 2010. https://doi.org/10.1002/cncr.24919.
46. Iyer JG, Blom A, Doumani R, et al. Response rates and durability of chemotherapy among 62 patients with metastatic Merkel cell carcinoma. Cancer Med 2016. https://doi.org/10.1002/cam4.815.
47. Kaufman HL, Russell J, Hamid O, et al. Avelumab in patients with chemotherapy-refractory metastatic Merkel cell carcinoma: a multicentre, single-group, open-label, phase 2 trial. Lancet Oncol 2016. https://doi.org/10.1016/S1470-2045(16)30364-3.
48. Kaufman HL, Russell JS, Hamid O, et al. Updated efficacy of avelumab in patients with previously treated metastatic Merkel cell carcinoma after $\geq$1 year of follow-up: JAVELIN Merkel 200, a phase 2 clinical trial. J Immunother Cancer 2018. https://doi.org/10.1186/s40425-017-0310-x.
49. Nghiem PT, Bhatia S, Lipson EJ, et al. PD-1 blockade with pembrolizumab in advanced merkel-cell carcinoma. N Engl J Med 2016. https://doi.org/10.1056/NEJMoa1603702.
50. Topalian SL, Bhatia S, Hollebecque A, et al. Non-comparative, open-label, multiple cohort, phase 1/2 study to evaluate nivolumab (NIVO) in patients with virus-associated tumors (CheckMate 358): efficacy and safety in Merkel cell carcinoma (MCC). Cancer Res 2017. https://doi.org/10.1158/1538-7445.AM2017-CT074.
51. Lipson EJ, Vincent JG, Loyo M, et al. PD-L1 expression in the Merkel cell carcinoma microenvironment: association with inflammation, Merkel cell polyomavirus, and overall survival. Cancer Immunol Res 2013;1(1):54–63.
52. Blackmon JT, Dhawan R, Viator TM, et al. Talimogene laherparepvec for regionally advanced Merkel cell carcinoma: a report of 2 cases. JAAD Case Rep 2017. https://doi.org/10.1016/j.jdcr.2017.02.003.
53. Nardi V, Song Y, Santamaria-Barria JA, et al. Activation of PI3K signaling in Merkel cell carcinoma. Clin Cancer Res 2012;18(5):1227–36.
54. Shiver MB, Mahmoud F, Gao L. Response to Idelalisib in a patient with stage IV Merkel-Cell carcinoma. N Engl J Med 2015. https://doi.org/10.1056/NEJMc1507446.
55. Davids M, Charlton A, Ng SS, et al. Response to a novel multitargeted tyrosine kinase inhibitor pazopanib in metastatic merkel cell carcinoma. J Clin Oncol 2009. https://doi.org/10.1200/JCO.2009.21.8149.
56. Rabinowits G, Lezcano C, Catalano PJ, et al. Cabozantinib in patients with advanced Merkel cell carcinoma. Oncologist 2018. https://doi.org/10.1634/theoncologist.2017-0552.
57. Samlowski WE, Moon J, Tuthill RJ, et al. A phase ii trial of imatinib mesylate in Merkel cell carcinoma (neuroendocrine carcinoma of the skin). Am J Clin Oncol 2010;33(5):495–9.

58. Loader DE, Feldmann R, Baumgartner M, et al. Clinical remission of Merkel cell carcinoma after treatment with imatinib. J Am Acad Dermatol 2013. https://doi.org/10.1016/j.jaad.2013.03.042.

59. Paulson KG, Carter JJ, Johnson LG, et al. Antibodies to merkel cell polyomavirus T antigen oncoproteins reflect tumor burden in Merkel cell carcinoma patients. Cancer Res 2010;70(21):8388–97.

60. Paulson KG, Lewis CW, Redman MW, et al. Viral oncoprotein antibodies as a marker for recurrence of Merkel cell carcinoma: a prospective validation study. Cancer 2017;123(8):1464–74.

61. Brewer JD, Shanafelt TD, Otley CC, et al. Chronic lymphocytic Leukemia is associated with decreased survival of patients with malignant melanoma and merkel cell carcinoma in a SEER population-based study. J Clin Oncol 2012;30(8):843–9.

62. Paulson KG, Iyer JG, Blom A, et al. Systemic immune suppression predicts diminished Merkel cell carcinoma–specific survival independent of stage. J Invest Dermatol 2013;133(3):642–6.

63. Andea AA, Coit DG, Amin B, et al. Merkel cell carcinoma: histologic features and prognosis. Cancer 2008. https://doi.org/10.1002/cncr.23874.

64. Fields RC, Busam KJ, Chou JF, et al. Five hundred patients with merkel cell carcinoma evaluated at a single institution. Ann Surg 2011. https://doi.org/10.1097/SLA.0b013e31822c5fc1.

65. Asioli S, Righi A, De Biase D, et al. Expression of p63 is the sole independent marker of aggressiveness in localised (stage I-II) Merkel cell carcinomas. Mod Pathol 2011. https://doi.org/10.1038/modpathol.2011.100.

66. Stetsenko GY, Malekirad J, Paulson KG, et al. P63 expression in merkel cell carcinoma predicts poorer survival yet may have limited clinical utility. Am J Clin Pathol 2013. https://doi.org/10.1309/AJCPE4PK6CTBNQJY.

67. Paulson KG, Iyer JG, Tegeder AR, et al. Transcriptome-wide studies of merkel cell carcinoma and validation of intratumoral cd8+ lymphocyte invasion as an independent predictor of survival. J Clin Oncol 2011. https://doi.org/10.1200/JCO.2010.30.6308.

68. Sihto H, Bohling T, Kavola H, et al. Tumor infiltrating immune cells and outcome of Merkel cell carcinoma: a population-based study. Clin Cancer Res 2012;18(10):2872–81.

Malignant Sweat Gland Tumors

Christine S. Ahn, MD, Omar P. Sangüeza, MD*

KEYWORDS

- Cutaneous • Porocarcinoma • Pilomatrixcarcinoma • Hidradenocarcinoma
- Cylindrocarcinoma

KEY POINTS

- The classification of malignant sweat gland neoplasms has undergone changes over time.
- Malignant sweat gland neoplasms have variable malignant potential, with some behaving as indolent tumors and others with high metastatic potential.
- Many of the sweat gland neoplasms have overlapping features but knowledge of the characteristic findings of these entities is important.

INTRODUCTION

The classification of adnexal tumors is regarded as one of the more confusing aspects of dermatopathology, because of its evolution over time. Several entities, originally thought to be derived from eccrine glands because of their location in nonapocrine sites of the body, have undergone alternate classification of authors, now considered to be apocrine in origin. Classification immunohistochemical staining has provided some clarification, such as the staining of certain sweat gland tumors with eccrine gland-associated monoclonal antibodies (EKH-5, EKH-6), which stains the eccrine secretory coil.

Eccrine carcinomas are particularly confusing to classify, because some tumors demonstrate heterogenous features that defy existing classification systems. In this review, sweat gland carcinomas are discussed, with a focus on key clinical and histopathologic features of each entity.

POROCARCINOMA
Clinical Features

Porocarcinoma, also known as eccrine porocarcinoma and malignant poroma, is a malignant tumor derived from the intraepidermal portion of the eccrine sweat duct.

Disclosure Statement: The authors have no commercial or financial conflicts of interest to disclose.
Department of Pathology, Wake Forest School of Medicine, Medical Center Boulevard, Winston Salem, NC 27157, USA
* Corresponding author.
E-mail address: osanguez@wakehealth.edu

It is typically seen in older patients, although there are reports of occurrence in all ages. There seems to be no gender nor racial predilection.[1] Lesions tend to occur on the legs in up to 60% of cases, particularly favoring the thigh and knee. Other sites of involvement include the head, neck, and trunk. Few reports in the literature describe rare cases of porocarcinoma occurring on unusual locations, such as the vulva, periungal soft tissue, and the eyelid.[2–4]

Porocarcinoma present as a solitary nodule or tumor, occasionally with verrucous epidermal changes and/or ulceration (**Fig. 1**). Most cases of porocarcinoma occur de novo and grow slowly or remain stable for several years. Because of the slow growth, lesions are often asymptomatic, which may contribute to a delay in diagnosis. Some studies estimate 30% to 50% of porocarcinoma arise from longstanding preexisting poroma. In these cases, lesions are characterized by rapid growth, ulceration, bleeding, or pain. In one review of 453 cases of porocarcinoma, the mean duration to presentation was more than 5 years, and 31% of cases were found to have concomitant metastases at the time of presentation, with nearby lymph nodes most commonly involved (58%), followed by visceral metastases to the lung (13%).[1] Because of the rarity of the neoplasm, there are no established therapeutic algorithms. However, the mainstay of treatment is surgical removal, achieved by wide local excision with histologic confirmation of tumor-free margins, which is curative in 70% to 80% of cases. The definitive role of sentinel lymph node biopsy is not fully understood, but may be indicated in the presence of certain risk factors, such as deep invasion (greater than 7 mm), high mitotic rate, and the presence of lymphovascular invasion.[5] More recently, there has been increasing evidence to support the use of Mohs micrographic surgery for removal of the tumor.[6,7] Chemotherapy and radiotherapy have been used with variable success, and are primarily used as adjunctive treatment of recurrent or metastatic disease.[8,9]

Histopathologic Features

On scanning magnification, porocarcinoma are large, asymmetric proliferations with classically malignant features, such as poor circumscription and an invasive growth pattern. Large areas of necrosis en masse are frequently observed in porocarcinoma, although this finding can also be seen in benign poromas. The surrounding stroma is scarce, and the dermis and subcutaneous tissue is filled with aggregates of cells with irregular borders and variable in size and shape (**Fig. 2**A). Similar to poromas, the tumor is composed of poroid and cuticular cells, although the poroid cells are the predominant neoplastic cells, with few cuticular cells seen around small ductal structures

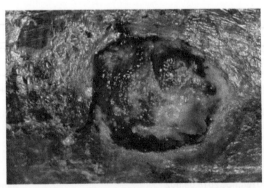

Fig. 1. Porocarcinoma. Ulcerated, friable tumor with areas of verrucous epidermal changes.

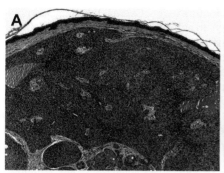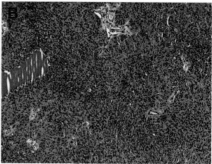

Fig. 2. Porocarcinoma. (*A*) Scanning view of a porocarcinoma with a dense proliferation of poroid cells and cuticle-lined ducts (hematoxylin-eosin, original magnification ×4). (*B*) Higher power of the same tumor shows scarce stroma and cellular atypia (hematoxylin-eosin, original magnification ×10).

(**Fig. 2**B). There are some cases that describe "giant cell porocarcinomas," which refers to porocarcinomas where the atypical cuticular cells are the predominant neoplastic cells.[10] Other unusual features that may be observed in porocarcinoma include clear cell changes, the presence of dendritic melanocytes, intralesional regions of malignant squamous differentiation, multinucleated neoplastic cells, and metaplastic or sarcomatoid transformation.[11,12]

Porocarcinoma are most commonly confused with invasive squamous cell carcinoma. Immunohistochemical markers helpful in diagnosing porocarcinoma include carcinoembryonic antigen (CEA) and cytokeratin (CK) 7; however, these markers can have variable expression in squamous cell carcinoma. CK19 may be a helpful marker in distinguishing porocarcinoma from squamous cell carcinoma, with a specificity of 82% in one study.[13]

TUBULAR CARCINOMA
Clinical Features

Primary cutaneous tubular carcinoma, also known as apocrine adenocarcinoma and apocrine tubular carcinoma, is a malignant apocrine neoplasm that typically arises in areas where there is a high density of apocrine glands, such as the axillae and groin, although cases have been reported in the eyelid, scalp, nipple, lip, and ear canal, and within preexisting nevus sebaceous.[14,15] They appear more frequently in women in the fourth to sixth decades of life. This entity presents as a solitary firm, subcutaneous, red to violaceous nodule that can sometimes seem adherent to the underlying tissue. Longstanding lesions may develop ulceration. Tubular carcinoma exhibits locally aggressive behavior, associated with high rates of local recurrence and potentially widespread metastases. In poorly differentiated apocrine adenocarcinomas, up to 50% of cases have had regional lymph node metastases at the time of presentation.[16] Distant metastases occur through lymphatic or hematogenous spread, and are most frequently observed in the liver, bone, lungs, brain, skin, and parotid gland. The treatment of choice is wide local excision with sentinel lymph node biopsy and possible adjuvant therapy with radiation or chemotherapy.[17]

Histopathologic Features

At scanning magnification, apocrine tubular carcinoma is a poorly circumscribed dermal-based tumor with little or no connection to the overlying epidermis, composed of a mixed pattern of tubular and ductal structures with. Overall, the epithelium predominates with a scarce surrounding stroma. In some lesions, a desmoplastic stroma or lymphoplasmacytic infiltrate may be seen between neoplastic ducts. In the superficial dermis, neoplastic tubules have a broader lumen, occasionally with intraluminal papillary projections. Foamy histiocytes and granular eosinophilic material may be seen within the lumina, along with decapitation secretion in the neoplastic ductal structures, and areas of tumor necrosis.[18] The size of the ducts and tubules decrease in the deeper levels of the dermis. Cases of poorly differentiated tubular carcinoma demonstrate less prominent apocrine features and decapitation secretion, and neoplastic cells have marked pleomorphism, prominent nucleoli, and numerous mitotic figures. Well-differentiated tubular carcinoma can sometimes be mistake for benign apocrine adenoma, which can lead to inadequate initial treatment. Increased expression of low-molecular-weight kininogen is observed in tumor cells, whereas luminal cells demonstrate increased expression of CEA, epithelial membrane antigen (EMA), and gross cystic disease fluid protein 15.[19]

AGGRESSIVE DIGITAL PAPILLARY CARCINOMA
Clinical Features

Papillary carcinoma, also described as aggressive digital papillary adenocarcinoma, is notable for its preferential location on the digits. Initially, papillary adenomas were distinguished from adenocarcinomas based on the degree of differentiation. However, Duke and colleagues[20] found that the histopathologic criteria initially proposed did not differentiate benign from malignant entities, because lesions previously designated as benign were found to subsequently metastasize. This group concluded that all lesions on this spectrum should be considered malignant, proposing the term "aggressive digital papillary adenocarcinoma."[21]

This entity occurs more frequently in men than in women and is most common in whites. It is typically seen on the volar surface of the digit or in the periungual region, although there are few reports of alternate locations, including the wrist and the heel. This neoplasm is seen mostly in adults in the fifth to seventh decades of life, with few reports of cases in children. Clinically, lesions present as a subcutaneous, firm nodule, often with overlying ulceration. The differential diagnosis may include paronychia or other cutaneous infections, and acquired digital fibrokeratoma. The mainstay of treatment is complete removal of the tumor, often involving amputation of the digit. However, despite complete removal, local recurrence rates of 16% to 50% and metastasis rates of 14% to 41% have been reported.[21,22] Distant metastases occur most commonly in the lung and lymph nodes. Additionally, metastatic spread has been observed in patients treated with wide local excision and amputation even in the absence of locally recurrent disease. Some authors have reported successful use of Mohs micrographic surgery as a digit-sparing alternative of treatment.[23]

Histopathologic Features

Papillary carcinoma are multinodular and usually poorly circumscribed tumors that extend from the dermis to the subcutis, typically with no connection with the epidermis (Fig. 3A). This lesion is infiltrative and perineural invasion is a common feature. The neoplasm is predominantly a solid neoplasm with focal areas of tubular structures and papillary projections. Cribriform patterns without epithelial papillations may also be observed in this entity. The solid component of the tumor consists of neoplastic cells with hyperchromatic and pleomorphic nuclei with small ductal structures. Papillary projections are lined by cuboidal or columnar cells with cytoplasmic projections

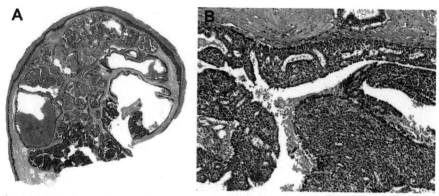

Fig. 3. Aggressive digital papillary carcinoma. (*A*) Scanning view of an aggressive digital papillary carcinoma with solid and cystic components, areas of cribriform pattern, tubular structures, and papillary projections (hematoxylin-eosin, original magnification ×1). (*B*) Higher power view of the solid components of the same tumor demonstrates neoplastic cells with hyperchromatic and pleomorphic nuclei and glandular lumina containing eosinophilic secretory material (hematoxylin-eosin, original magnification ×10).

and varying degrees of atypia (**Fig. 3**B). Additional features of papillary carcinoma include necrosis within the neoplastic aggregates, squamous eddies around ductal structures, areas of sebaceous differentiation, a lymphoplasmacytic infiltrate, and neoplastic cells within vascular or lymphatic structures.[24]

Immunohistochemical studies demonstrate positivity for S-100 in the cytoplasm of some neoplastic cells and CEA along the luminal cells of papillae and tubular structures.[24]

ADENOID CYSTIC CARCINOMA
Clinical Features

Adenoid cystic carcinoma (ACC) are malignant neoplasms that are commonly described in the salivary glands and other organs, such as the trachea, breast, Bartholin glands, and prostate. Primary cutaneous ACC was first described in 1975.[25] This lesion is observed in adults, affecting men and women equally. The most common location is the scalp, although lesions on the face, trunk, and extremities have been described. Lesions are often asymptomatic with nonspecific clinical features, usually presenting as a solitary subcutaneous nodule or multiple nodules coalescing into a plaque. Patients with primary cutaneous ACC are at significantly higher risk of lymphohematopoietic malignancy.[26] In contrast to salivary or lacrimal gland ACC, primary cutaneous ACC tends to follow a more indolent course. Perineural invasion is not uncommon, and seems to be associated with local recurrence.[27]

Histopathologic Features

Similar to other malignant sweat gland neoplasms described, ACC are poorly circumscribed tumors situated in the dermis and often extending into the subcutaneous tissue (**Fig. 4**A). The tumor is composed of epithelial collections of basaloid cells in alternating solid and cribriform areas. Epithelial cells are basophilic, monomorphous, with hyperchromatic nuclei. Most cutaneous ACC exhibit low-grade cytologic atypia and low mitotic activity. The cribriform areas represent pseudoglandular adenoid spaces that form as a result of necrosis of neoplastic cells. They contain mucin, cell

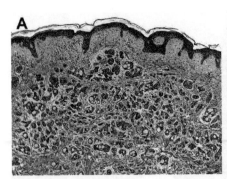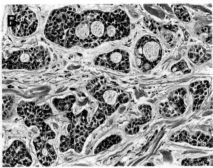

Fig. 4. Adenoid cystic carcinoma. (*A*) Scanning view of an adenoid cystic carcinoma with a cribriform pattern with ducts and duct-like spaces filled with mucin (hematoxylin-eosin, original magnification ×4). (*B*) Higher power view of epithelial islands with a cribriform pattern (hematoxylin-eosin, original magnification ×20).

basement membrane material, and cellular debris (**Fig. 4**B). True ductal structures are also present, in smaller number, in ACC, which are characterized by a lining of cuboidal cells and a peripheral layer of myoepithelial cells. Decapitation secretion is observed within the ducts, and ultrastructural studies demonstrate the presence of microvilli within the lumen.[28]

In a study of the immunohistochemical and molecular features of primary cutaneous ACC, vimentin was diffusely positive in 57% of cutaneous ACC and CK15 was diffusely positive in 36%. In contrast, all salivary ACCs were negative or focally positive and thus these stains may help differentiate between primary cutaneous and salivary gland ACCs.[29]

CRIBRIFORM CARCINOMA
Clinical Features

Cribriform carcinoma is a rare cutaneous adenocarcinoma exhibiting apocrine differentiation. First described in 1998 by Requena and colleagues,[30] this malignant sweat gland neoplasm is observed in young to middle-aged adults. Women are more frequently affected than men, and the average age at the time of diagnosis is 47 years.[31] The most common locations are the upper and lower extremities, with few reports on the head and trunk. Clinically, lesions present with nonspecific features, usually as slow-growing, solitary, subcutaneous nodules that feel firmly attached to underlying tissue. The clinical differential diagnosis includes an inflamed epidermal inclusion cyst or dermatofibroma.

Primary cutaneous cribriform carcinoma is considered a low-grade malignancy, with no reports of local recurrence or metastases after complete resection of the lesion.[31]

Histopathologic Features

The most distinct feature of this tumor is the cribriform pattern with nests of epithelial islands surrounded by a desmoplastic stroma. Cribriform carcinoma may not exhibit typical features of malignant neoplasms; it is often a well-circumscribed, nonencapsulated dermal nodule (**Fig. 5**A). There is usually no connection to the overlying epidermis, and cribriform and tubular structures are the major architectural patterns.[32] The cribriform areas can consist of small sieve-like spaces, or larger cystic spaces

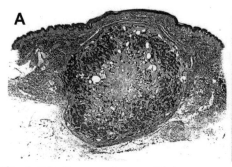
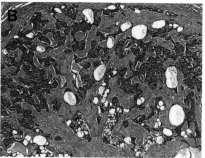

Fig. 5. Cribriform carcinoma. (*A*) Low-power view shows a well-circumscribed dermal nodule composed of small sieve-like spaces (hematoxylin-eosin, original magnification ×10). (*B*) Higher power view shows interconnected epithelioid cells set in a desmoplastic stroma (hematoxylin-eosin, original magnification ×15).

lined by flattened epithelial cells. In some cases, the cribriform pattern may not predominate and the neoplasm can appear largely solid, with only focal cribriform areas.[31] The epithelial component consists of interconnected epithelioid cells with pleomorphic and polygonal nuclei (**Fig. 5**B). Focal areas of necrosis and necrosis en masse may be observed. In some cases, a second population of solid epithelial cells are seen, with a distinct cytomorphology, with larger and paler nuclei, abundant eosinophilic cytoplasm, and with infiltrative features at the periphery of the tumor with evidence of stromal retraction. Lymphovascular or perineural invasion is not a feature of this entity.

The desmoplastic stroma of cribriform carcinoma is scarce and composed of fibrillary collagen and fibroblasts. Some areas may appear myxoid, although this is not a characteristic feature. A lymphoplasmacytic perivascular infiltrate or nodular lymphoid aggregates can be seen at the periphery of the tumor.

The main differential diagnosis for cribriform carcinoma is ACC, which is characterized by epithelial islands of basaloid cells and small cyst-like spaces. However, the spaces are usually larger in ACC, aggregates of neoplastic basaloid cells are less likely to be interconnected, and neurotropism is much more frequently observed. Other entities that can share similar features include primary cutaneous secretory carcinoma and metastatic carcinoma.[32]

There are few reports of the use of immunohistochemical studies in cribriform carcinoma. Neoplastic cells usually express CKs (AE1/AE3, CAM 5/2, CK5/6, CK7), EMA, CEA, S100, and CD117. They are usually nonreactive for CK20 and SMA.[32]

APOCRINE HIDRADENOCARCINOMA
Clinical Features

Apocrine hidradenocarcinoma is an entity that has been reported under numerous designations, including clear cell hidradenocarcinoma, clear cell malignant acrospiroma, nodular hidroadenocarcinoma, and malignant eccrine acrospiroma, among others. This is a rare and aggressive malignancy, observed slightly more frequently in men than in women and primarily in adults. Clinically, this neoplasm presents as an asymptomatic subcutaneous red to violaceous nodule and tends to favor the face, hands, and feet, although they can occur anywhere. The lesion is slow-growing, often leading to several years' duration before seeking treatment in most case reports. In instances of sudden rapid growth, the possibility of malignant transformation of a preexisting apocrine hidradenoma is considered.[33] The mainstay of treatment of local disease is surgical excision, but based on limited data, there is a high rate of local recurrence, metastasis, and poor outcomes associated with this entity, with up to 60% of patients presenting with metastases within the first 2 years.[34]

Histopathologic Features

Apocrine hidradenocarcinoma are multilobulated tumors within the dermis, extending in the subcutis. The overall architecture is asymmetric with aggregates of neoplastic cells that vary in shape and size (**Fig. 6**A). Tubular formation is observed in most lesions, but may be only a focal finding in some. The overlying epidermis is typically uninvolved, although ulceration may be present. Occasional connection between the tumor and follicular infundibula is seen.

The neoplastic cells of apocrine hidradenocarcinoma can appear as clear or pale cells, squamous, polygonal, oncocytoid, or mucinous. The clear or pale appearance is caused by abundant glycogen within the cytoplasm (**Fig. 6**B), whereas squamous cells have an eosinophilic and granular cytoplasm and may form squamous eddies. The stroma of this tumor is sclerotic, although a desmoplastic stroma can be seen in the deeper portions of the neoplasm, imparting a sarcomatoid appearance.

Malignant hidradenocarcinoma is distinguished from benign hidradenoma by its poor circumscription, infiltrative growth pattern, deep extension, necrosis, perineural invasion, vascular invasion, nuclear pleomorphism, or increased mitotic figures.[35,36]

MALIGNANT MIXED TUMOR OF THE SKIN
Clinical Features

Malignant mixed tumor of the skin, also known as malignant chondroid syringoma, are uncommon, with less than 50 cases described in the literature. The nomenclature is derived from the fact that this neoplasm is a tumor of epithelial and mesenchymal origin.[37] It can occur de novo or arise within a preexisting benign chondroid syringoma. Clinically, lesions are nonspecific, presenting as a subcutaneous nodule with possible overlying ulceration and firm attachment to underlying tissue. It is seen more often in women than in men, and typically in adults. In contrast to its benign counterpart, malignant mixed tumors are usually found on the extremities, with the hands and feet being frequent locations. In contrast, mixed tumors of the skin are most commonly observed on the face and scalp.

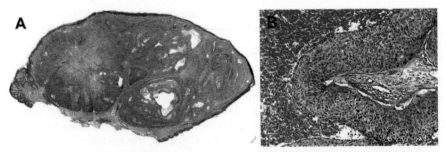

Fig. 6. Apocrine hidradenocarcinoma. (*A*) Scanning view of an apocrine hidradenocarcinoma with an infiltrative, lobular proliferation in the dermis and subcutis with evidence of necrosis (hematoxylin-eosin, original magnification ×1). (*B*) Higher power view of atypical cells with a clear appearance (hematoxylin-eosin, original magnification ×10).

The mainstay of treatment of malignant mixed tumor of the skin is wide local excision. However, there are rare reports of long-term distant and lymph node metastases after complete removal.[38,39]

Histopathologic Features

At scanning magnification, malignant mixed tumors are asymmetric proliferations within the dermis and infiltrating into the subcutaneous tissue (**Fig. 7**A). The tumor is poorly circumscribed and can infiltrate underlying muscle and bone. It is composed of an epithelial and mesenchymal component with mucin deposition. Within the epithelial component, small tubules and ducts are present, which are similar to the tubular formations seen in benign mixed tumors. The tubules and ducts appear lined by columnar cells, with evidence of decapitation secretion within the lumina (**Fig. 7**B). Thus, malignant mixed tumors are thought to show apocrine differentiation. The epithelial component can also lack ductal formation, and consist of solid aggregates of neoplastic cells, occasionally with isolated groups or cords of epithelial cells with a plasmacytoid or polygonal appearance. The epithelial cells are atypical with hyperchromatic nuclei and abundant mitotic figures, with occasional areas of necrosis. The mesenchymal component of this neoplasm is largely myxoid, although chondroid matrix or osteoid areas can be present (**Fig. 7**C).

Immunohistochemical studies are not always helpful in establishing the diagnosis, because benign chondroid syringoma may express similar profiles as malignant counterparts, including S100 and CK7, with negative expression of p63, EMA, CK5/6, and calponin 7.[37]

SYRINGOID CARCINOMA
Clinical Features

Syringoid carcinoma, first designated as an eccrine epithelioma, but also referred to as malignant syringoma, syringoid eccrine carcinoma, basal cell epithelioma with eccrine differentiation, and sclerosing syringoma, is a rare malignant neoplasm that is characterized by its similar histopathologic appearance to syringoma. This tumor is observed in men and women equally and presents on the face and scalp most frequently.[40] They are often slow-growing, and present as tender nodules or plaques. Alopecia is associated with syringoid carcinoma within lesions on hair-bearing sites. Overlying epidermal ulceration is a rare finding, usually observed in enlarging lesions.

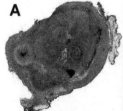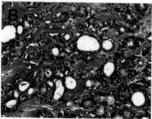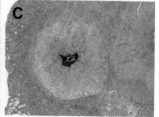

Fig. 7. Malignant mixed tumor of the skin. (*A*) Scanning view shows a poorly circumscribed dermal tumor with epithelial tumor islands and chondroid matrix areas (hematoxylin-eosin, original magnification ×1). (*B*) High power view of epithelial cords with cuticle-lined ducts (hematoxylin-eosin, original magnification ×20). (*C*) Focal chondroid regions within the mesenchymal component of the neoplasm (hematoxylin-eosin, original magnification ×2).

Syringoid carcinoma is a locally invasive tumor and is associated with local recurrences. Lymph node and distant metastases are exceedingly uncommon in this entity.[40]

Histopathologic Features

Syringoid carcinoma can show a variety of histologic features, but is characterized by the presence of ductal structures and small cysts throughout the dermis and often infiltrating into the subcutaneous tissue (**Fig. 8**A). The ductal structures exhibit the "tadpole" or "paisley-tie" appearance that is characteristic of syringoma, with lumina lined by an eosinophilic cuticle. Cysts are present in the upper dermis and may resemble small infundibular cysts or cysts of the distal portion of the eccrine or apocrine duct (**Fig. 8**B). Despite sharing many features, syringoid carcinoma is distinguished from its benign counterpart by the infiltrative growth pattern into adjacent tissue, cellularity, anaplasia, and by the presence of cords of neoplastic cells at distant sites. Additional distinctive features of syringoid carcinoma are destruction of adnexal structures and perineural infiltration in deeper areas of the tumor. The stroma is fibrotic or sclerotic, and lymphocytic infiltrates can be present in lymphoid aggregates throughout the lesion. As observed in the clear cell variant of syringoma, syringoid carcinoma can also have clear cells lining the neoplastic ductal structures.

Important differential diagnoses to consider with syringoid carcinoma are microcystic adnexal carcinoma (MAC), morpheaform basal cell carcinoma, syringoma, desmoplastic trichoepithelioma, or trichoadenoma, particularly if a superficial biopsy is performed. Immunohistochemical studies are of limited value in syringoid carcinoma, because the immunophenotype of this entity is not specific and often inconsistent. However, CK and CEA are consistently positive, although other antigens, such as EMA, Ber-EP4, ER, and PR have also been reported to be positive.[41]

CYLINDROCARCINOMA
Clinical Features

This rare neoplasm was first described in 1929 by Wiedman. Cylindrocarcinomas typically occur on the scalp, and the presence of multiple cylindromas seems to be the most common predisposing factor for developing cylindrocarcinoma.[42] Like other sweat gland neoplasms, this tumor lacks distinctive clinical features, but the most common presentation is a nodule of rapid growth arising in patients with multiple

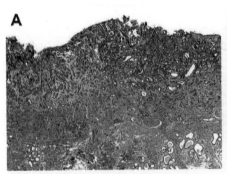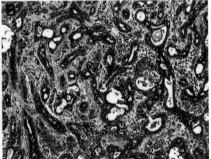

Fig. 8. Syringoid carcinoma. (A) Low-power view of syringoid carcinoma composed of small cysts and ductal structures infiltrating into the subcutaneous tissue (hematoxylin-eosin, original magnification ×2). (B) High power view of ductal structures lined by an eosinophilic cuticle with cords of neoplastic cells (hematoxylin-eosin, original magnification ×10).

long-standing cylindromas. The sudden rapid growth often leads to ulceration of the overlying skin. This neoplasm is highly aggressive, with distant metastases frequently reported.[43]

Histopathologic Features

Cylindrocarcinomas can look strikingly similar to cylindromas on low magnification, with dense aggregates of basaloid cells arranged in a jigsaw puzzle.[42] Benign and malignant components are often present in the same lesion. In cylindrocarcinoma, the neoplastic aggregates show variability in shape and size, and large areas of necrosis en masse are characteristic (**Fig. 9**). The overall architecture of the neoplasm can help differentiate from cylindromas, with a deep infiltrative growth pattern more consistent with cylindrocarcinoma. Immunohistochemical studies show variation in staining patterns, but there seems to be expression of vimentin and CK in epithelial cells.[42]

SPIRADENOCARCINOMA
Clinical Features

Spiradenocarcinomas, also known as malignant eccrine spiradenomas, are rare cutaneous adnexal neoplasms that arise from longstanding benign spiradenomas. A history of trauma to preexisting spiradenoma has also been reported. Rarely, they are seen in the setting of Brooke-Spiegler syndrome. They are seen in men and women equally, and usually observed in adults. The most common locations are the extremities, although there are reports of occurrences on the face, scalp, and chest. The most common symptoms are accelerated growth, pain, and ulceration. They are associated with aggressive behavior, although recent literature has suggested that lesions with low-grade morphologic features are associated with a more favorable clinical course.[44] Because of the rarity of the disease, there is no established treatment of spiradenocarcinoma, but radical excision is considered the mainstay of treatment. There are few reports of Mohs micrographic surgery used successfully for the treatment of spiradenocarcinoma.[45]

Histopathologic Features

In well-differentiated lesions, spiradenocarcinoma can share the key features of spiradenomas, which consists of dermal basaloid islands with multiple cuticle-lined ducts

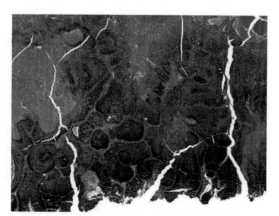

Fig. 9. Cylindrocarcinoma. Scanning view of a cylindrocarcinoma demonstrating focal areas of benign-appearing cylindroma along with large areas of necrosis (hematoxylin-eosin, original magnification ×2).

sprinkled with lymphocytes. In one study, all spiradenocarcinomas contained a component of a benign eccrine spiradenoma, which were composed of lobular, nested, and trabecular growth patterns and low mitotic activity. Malignant tumors are distinguished from spiradenoma by the asymmetric architecture and poorly circumscribed nature of the lesion, although most cases can still appear well circumscribed (**Fig. 10**A). The presence of necrosis and ectatic blood vessels with or without hemorrhage may be a diagnostic clue in this malignant neoplasm.[46] The epithelial cells demonstrate variability in shape and size, and large areas of necrosis en masse are frequently seen (**Fig. 10**B). Cords of neoplastic cells are seen infiltrating at the periphery of the tumor. Poorly differentiated spiradenocarcinoma are most distinct from spiradenoma, and the diagnosis often depends on the presence of focal areas resembling a spiradenoma. These lesions can appear anaplastic and sarcomatous. Lymphovascular invasion is not usually observed, and focal perineural invasion is rarely seen.[46]

Most spiradenocarcinoma stain positively for CK5 to CK7, and tumor protein p53 in up to 90% of cases in one study.[44]

MUCINOUS CARCINOMA
Clinical Features

Primary cutaneous mucinous carcinoma are rare low-grade malignant neoplasms thought to be of eccrine origin. Most mucinous carcinomas involving the skin are metastatic from breast, gastrointestinal tract, salivary glands, lacrimal glands, nasal sinuses, bronchi, or ovaries. One of the greatest challenges in diagnosing primary cutaneous mucinous carcinoma is differentiating this entity from metastatic disease. Both entities are nearly identical with similar gross and histologic features.[47] Primary cutaneous mucinous carcinoma is seen in adults and affects men more than women. It occurs more frequently in white patients. The most common location is the head, particularly on the eyelids, followed by the face, neck, and scalp. Less often, lesions can occur on the axilla, chest, abdomen, legs, and perianal region. Primary cutaneous mucinous carcinoma presents as a solitary skin-colored nodule, although it can appear bluish gray or red. Ulceration is often seen with growth, and lesions on the scalp may have associated alopecia. This neoplasm generally demonstrates low metastatic potential, and local recurrences are high in some studies but it is thought to be

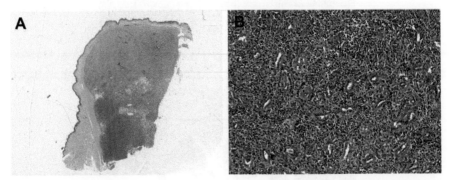

Fig. 10. Spiradenocarcinoma. (*A*) Scanning view of a spiradenocarcinoma with a dense proliferation of a dermal tumor with infiltrative growth (hematoxylin-eosin, original magnification ×1). (*B*) High-power view of basaloid islands with atypical neoplastic cells with marked atypia and pleomorphism (hematoxylin-eosin, original magnification ×10).

caused by incomplete resection. There is no standard of care for the surgical treatment of mucinous carcinoma, but may include wide local excision, regional lymph node dissection, and Mohs micrographic surgery.[48]

Histopathologic Features

On histology, mucinous carcinoma is characterized by aggregates of neoplastic cells within pools of mucin, separated by thin fibrous septae (**Fig. 11**A). The epithelial cells are arranged in clusters and demonstrate variation in size and shape but are typically small in size. Tumor cells are strongly positive for CK7, and negative for CK20.[48] Between epithelial components, tubular structures may be present. At the periphery of the epithelial collections or within the lumina of tubules, decapitation secretion may be observed although is not a constant feature of this entity (**Fig. 11**B). Different patterns may be observed focally within primary cutaneous mucinous carcinoma, including adenoid-cystic, cribriform, papillary, cystic, and solid. Perineural invasion and lymphocytic infiltration by neoplastic cells may be observed.

Primary cutaneous mucinous carcinoma can also demonstrate neuroendocrine differentiation, which stains positively for CK7, EMA, and hormone receptors. Neuroendocrine differentiation is highlighted with markers, such as chromogranin, synaptophysin, or neuron-specific enolase.[49] Additionally, to help differentiate between primary lesions and metastases, the presence of in situ components in focal areas of the lesion is highlighted with immunohistochemical stains with smooth muscle markers, such as smooth muscle actin, p63, and calponin, which stain the peripheral layer of myoepithelial cells around the neoplastic aggregates. The presence of this staining pattern favors the diagnosis of primary cutaneous mucinous carcinoma over a cutaneous metastasis from a distant site.

POLYMORPHOUS SWEAT GLAND CARCINOMA
Clinical Features

Polymorphous sweat gland carcinoma is a rare neoplasm, with only 12 cases described in the literature. The lesion demonstrates a predilection for the extremities and is often misdiagnosed as a dermatofibroma or cyst. Based on few available reports, it seems to occur in middle aged to older patients, and affects men and women equally. In most case reports, patients present with an asymptomatic nodule after a

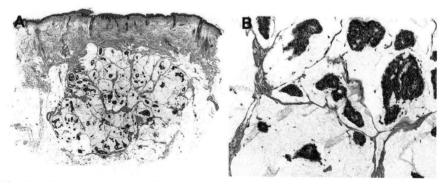

Fig. 11. Mucinous carcinoma. (*A*) Scanning view of mucinous carcinoma with islands of epithelial neoplastic cells within lakes of mucin in the dermis and subcutis (hematoxylin-eosin, original magnification ×1). (*B*) Higher power view of atypical epithelial cells arranged in clusters separated by thin fibrous septae (hematoxylin-eosin, original magnification ×10).

prolonged clinical course. It is characterized by variegate histopathologic findings and low-grade clinical behavior.[50]

Histopathologic Features

Polymorphous sweat gland carcinoma is characterized histologically by a dermal proliferation of epithelial aggregates in a combination of different patterns, including solid areas, tubular structures, papillary formations, and cylindromatous and adenoid-cystic areas (**Fig. 12**A). These various growth patterns can appear admixed within the same tumor, although the most common patterns are the cribriform or adenoid cystic pattern. Tumor cells are variable, ranging from round to polygonal with large prominent nucleoli and scattered mitotic figures. The epidermis is uninvolved, and tumors tend to infiltrate the full thickness of the dermis into the subcutaneous tissue. Surrounding hemorrhage, hyalinization, myxoid changes, and cystic areas are observed in the stroma (**Fig. 12**B).

On immunohistochemistry, this entity stains positively for CKAE1/3, CK5/6, p40, p63, and p16.[51]

MICROCYSTIC ADNEXAL CARCINOMA
Clinical Features

MAC is an uncommon, locally aggressive adnexal neoplasm. It may be an underdiagnosed entity caused by shared clinical and histologic features with other cutaneous neoplasms.[52] MAC affects men and women equally and can occur in a wide range of ages from the first to eighth decades of life. It is seen more frequently in white persons, and favors the periorbital and nasolabial regions. Less commonly, they are found on the nipple, axilla, vulva, hands, tongue, and extremities. It presents as a solitary nodule or firm plaque. On hair-bearing sites, such as the scalp, it can simulate a scarring alopecia.[52] On the lip, the lesion can feel indurated because of extension into the mucosa, and can lead to paresthesia of the involved lip because of neural involvement.

MAC is an indolent, infiltrative tumor with a propensity for perineural invasion. There are rare reports of lymph node metastases but typically it invades local structures. Mohs micrographic surgery has come to the forefront of treatment, thought to be preferable to standard surgical excision because of poorly defined clinical margins,

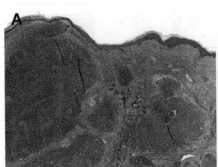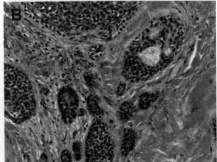

Fig. 12. Polymorphous sweat gland carcinoma. (*A*) Low-power view of polymorphous sweat gland carcinoma with a predominantly cribriform pattern (hematoxylin-eosin, original magnification ×2). (*B*) Higher power view of neoplastic cells with surrounding hyalinized stroma (hematoxylin-eosin, original magnification ×40).

perineural invasion, and location on the face. Other treatment options include wide excision and radiation.[53]

Histopathologic Features

MAC demonstrate features of eccrine and follicular differentiation. It is primarily a dermal tumor, organized in a layered manner. In the superficial part of the tumor, there are cystic keratinized structures that resemble milia cysts and small islands or cords of epithelium with ductal differentiation.[53] Within this portion of the tumor, calcification may be present within the keratinous cysts. In the center of the lesion, there are aggregates of pale or eosinophilic cells with variable shape and size. In the deep portion of the tumor, smaller nests and strands of neoplastic cells are present surrounded by a hyalinized stroma. Tubular structures are present, lined with epithelial cells and containing eosinophilic material and occasionally demonstrating decapitation secretion (**Fig. 13**).

The epithelial component predominates over the stroma in MAC, which is sclerotic with thickened collagen. Less common histopathologic findings of MAC include a peripheral syringomatous proliferation and scattered inflammatory infiltrates with eosinophils.

The differential diagnosis of MAC includes syringoma, syringoid carcinoma, and desmoplastic trichoepithelioma. The distinction between these entities is particularly challenging when superficial biopsy specimens are obtained. In desmoplastic trichoepithelioma, cords of neoplastic cells with surrounding eosinophilic collagen can appear similar to those of MAC. However, the epithelial cords of desmoplastic trichoepithelioma are basaloid, whereas in MAC they appear more eosinophilic. Although the immunohistochemical profile of MAC is not specific, numerous stains are used to help distinguish from infiltrative basal cell carcinoma and desmoplastic trichoepithelioma.[53]

SECRETORY CARCINOMA OF THE SKIN
Clinical Features

Secretory carcinoma of the skin is a rare neoplasm with only few reports to date. It appears as a solitary dermal or subcutaneous nodule and has most frequently been observed in the axillae. It affects females more often and is associated with an ETV6-NTRK3 translocation, which is a characteristic finding of secretory breast carcinoma and mammary analogue secretory carcinoma.[54]

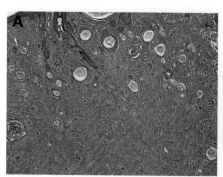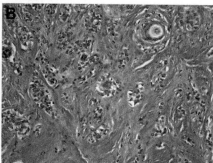

Fig. 13. Microcystic adnexal carcinoma. (*A*) Low-power view of MAC (hematoxylin-eosin, original magnification ×1). (*B*) Higher power view showing infiltrative growth pattern and poorly defined borders (hematoxylin-eosin, original magnification ×20).

Histopathologic Features

At scanning magnification, secretory carcinoma of the skin is poorly circumscribed and is composed of dense neoplastic aggregates involving the entire dermis and infiltrating into the subcutaneous tissue. There are intraductal and invasive components composed of aggregates of epithelial cells with bland nuclei and lumina containing bubbly eosinophilic secretion. Tumor cells are arranged in different growth patterns ranging from microcystic, tubular, solid, to papillary. Perineural or intravascular involvement has not been observed in the cases reported. Immunohistochemical staining demonstrates positive staining of tumor cells with S100, mammaglobin, and CK7. Less consistently positive markers are CAM5.2, CK19, and EMA, whereas tumor cells are negative for p63 and SMA expression.[54]

PRIMARY CUTANEOUS SIGNET RING CELL CARCINOMA
Clinical Features

Signet ring cell carcinoma or primary cutaneous histiocytoid carcinoma is a rare neoplasm that is typically located on the eyelids of adults. In a review of 39 cases, there was a male predominance, and most lesions were located on the eyelids, followed by the axillae. Clinically, lesions present as diffuse thickening of the involved eyelid or a nodule or induration in the axillae. Treatment options include surgical removal, which may be followed by adjuvant and maintenance chemotherapy.[55–57]

Histopathologic Features

The histologic findings of this entity are consistent across reported cases. The tumor is located within the dermis, sparing the overlying epidermis, and composed of a dense infiltration of neoplastic cells arranged in single cells, small strands, or small islands invading the dermis and subcutaneous tissue.[55] The individual cells characteristically form a single-file pattern and occasionally may form an intracellular lumen. They also feature large hyperchromatic nuclei and ample cytoplasm, and most demonstrate a signet-ring appearance, featuring spindle-shaped, eccentric and hyperchromatic nuclei, prominent nucleoli, and a large cytoplasmic vacuole. Immunohistochemical staining reveals positive staining for EMA, CK7, and gross cystic disease fluid protein-15.[55]

REFERENCES

1. Salih AM, Kakamad FH, Baba HO, et al. Porocarcinoma; presentation and management, a meta-analysis of 453 cases. Ann Med Surg (Lond) 2017;20:74–9.
2. Chua PY, Cornish KS, Stenhouse G, et al. A rare case of eccrine porocarcinoma of the eyelid. Semin Ophthalmol 2015;30(5–6):443–5.
3. Palleschi GM, Dragoni F, Urso C. Subungual eccrine porocarcinoma: rare but possible. Dermatol Surg 2017;43(7):995–6.
4. Fujimine-Sato A, Toyoshima M, Shigeta S, et al. Eccrine porocarcinoma of the vulva: a case report and review of the literature. J Med Case Rep 2016;10(1):319.
5. Vaz Salgado MA, García CG, Lopez Martin JA. Porocarcinoma: clinical evolution. Dermatol Surg 2010;36(2):264–7.
6. Nazemi A, Higgins S, Swift R, et al. Eccrine porocarcinoma: new insights and a systematic review of the literature. Dermatol Surg 2018;44(10):1247–61.
7. Tolkachjov SN, Hocker TL, Camilleri MJ, et al. Treatment of porocarcinoma with Mohs micrographic surgery: the Mayo Clinic experience. Dermatol Surg 2016;42(6):745–50.

8. de Bree E, Volalakis E, Tsetis D. Treatment of advanced malignant eccrine poroma with locoregional chemotherapy. Br J Dermatol 2005;152(5):1051–5.
9. Godillot C, Boulinguez S, Riffaud L. Complete response of a metastatic porocarcinoma treated with paclitaxel, cetuximab and radiotherapy. Eur J Cancer 2018; 90:142–5.
10. Snow SN, Reizner GT. Eccrine porocarcinoma of the face. J Am Acad Dermatol 1992;27:306–11.
11. D'Amato MS, Patterson RH, Guccion JG, et al. Porocarcinoma of the heel. A case report with unusual histologic features. Cancer 1996;78(4):751–7.
12. Mahomed F, Blok J, Grayson W. The squamous variant of eccrine porocarcinoma: a clinicopathological study of 21 cases. J Clin Pathol 2008;61(3):361–5.
13. Mahalingam M, Richards JE, Selim MA, et al. An immunohistochemical comparison of cytokeratin 7, cytokeratin 15, cytokeratin 19, CAM 5.2, carcinoembryonic antigen, and nestin in differentiating porocarcinoma from squamous cell carcinoma. Hum Pathol 2012;43(8):1265–72.
14. Llamas-Velasco M, Requena L, Podda M, et al. Apocrine intraductal carcinoma in situ in nevus sebaceus: two case reports. J Cutan Pathol 2014;41:944–9.
15. Pagano Boza C, Vigo R, Premoli JE, et al. A case report of a primary apocrine adenocarcinoma of the eyelid with literature review. Orbit 2018;1–4 [Epub ahead of print].
16. Chamberlain RS, Huber K, White JC, et al. Apocrine gland carcinoma of the axilla: review of the literature and recommendations for treatment. Am J Clin Oncol 1999;22:131–5.
17. Tolkachjov SN, Brewer JD, Bridges AG. Apocrine axillary adenocarcinoma: an aggressive adnexal tumor in middle-age individuals. Dermatol Surg 2018;44(6): 876–8.
18. Kathrotiya PR, Bridge AT, Warren SJ, et al. Primary apocrine adenocarcinoma of the axilla. Cutis 2015;95(5):271–4, 281.
19. Kim HK, Chung KI, Park BY, et al. Primary apocrine carcinoma of scalp: report of primary scalp cutaneous apocrine carcinoma indistinguishable from cutaneous metastasis of breast carcinoma. J Plast Reconstr Aesthet Surg 2012;65(3):e67–70.
20. Duke WH, Sherrod TT, Lupton GP. Aggressive digital papillary adenocarcinoma (aggressive digital papillary adenoma and adenocarcinoma revisited). Am J Surg Pathol 2000;24:775–84.
21. Kao GF, Helwig EB, Graham JH. Aggressive digital papillary adenoma and adenocarcinoma. A clinicopathologic study of 57 patients with histochemical, immunopathological and ultrastructural observations. J Cutan Pathol 1987;14: 129–76.
22. Suchak R, Wang WL, Prieto VG, et al. Cutaneous digital papillary adenocarcinoma: a clinicopathologic study of 31 cases of a rare neoplasm with new observations. Am J Surg Pathol 2012;36:1883–91.
23. Rismiller K, Knackstedt TJ. Aggressive digital papillary adenocarcinoma: population-based analysis of incidence, demographics, treatment, and outcomes. Dermatol Surg 2018;44(7):911–7.
24. Ceballos PI, Penneys NS, Acosta R. Aggressive digital papillary adenocarcinoma. J Am Acad Dermatol 1990;23:331–4.
25. Boggio R. Adenoid cystic carcinoma of the scalp. Arch Dermatol 1975;111: 793–4.
26. Dores GM, Huycke MM, Devesa SS, et al. Primary cutaneous adenoid cystic carcinoma in the United States: incidence, survival, and associated cancers, 1976 to 2005. J Am Acad Dermatol 2010;63:71–8.

27. Morrison AO, Gardner JM, Goldsmith SM, et al. Primary cutaneous adenoid cystic carcinoma of the scalp with p16 expression: a case report and review of the literature. Am J Dermatopathol 2014;36(9):e163–6.

28. Van der Kwast TH, Vuzevski VD, Ramaekers F, et al. Primary cutaneous adenoid cystic carcinoma: case report, immunohistochemistry, and review of the literature. Br J Dermatol 1988;118:567–78.

29. North JP, McCalmont TH, Fehr A, et al. Detection of MYB alterations and other immunohistochemical markers in primary cutaneous adenoid cystic carcinoma. Am J Surg Pathol 2015;39(10):1347–56.

30. Requena L, Kiryu H, Ackerman AB. Cribriform carcinoma. In: Requena L, Sangüeza O, editors. Neoplasm with apocrine differentiation. Philadelphia: Lippincott-Raven; 1998. p. 879–905.

31. Arps DP, Chan MP, Patel RM, et al. Primary cutaneous cribriform carcinoma: report of six cases with clinicopathologic data and immunohistochemical profile. J Cutan Pathol 2015;42(6):379–87.

32. Wu JD, Changchien CH, Liao KS. Primary cutaneous cribriform apocrine carcinoma: case report and literature review. Indian J Dermatol Venereol Leprol 2018;84:569–72.

33. Hernández-Pérez E, Cestoni-Parducci R. Nodular hidradenoma and hidradenocarcinoma. A 10-year review. J Am Acad Dermatol 1985;12:15–20.

34. Miller DH, Peterson JL, Buskirk SJ, et al. Management of metastatic apocrine hidradenocarcinoma with chemotherapy and radiation. Rare Tumors 2015;7(3): 6082.

35. Chan CM, Stewart BD2, Gibbs CP Jr. Hidradenocarcinoma of the finger: a rare tumor, mimicking a giant cell tumor of the tendon sheath. J Hand Surg Eur Vol 2016;41(9):1001–3.

36. Kazakov DV, Ivan D, Kutzner H, et al. Cutaneous hidradenocarcinoma: a clinicopathological, immunohistochemical, and molecular biologic study of 14 cases, including Her2/neu gene expression/amplification, TP53 gene mutation analysis, and t(11;19) translocation. Am J Dermatopathol 2009;31(3):236–47.

37. Lal K, Morrell TJ, Cunningham M, et al. A case of a malignant cutaneous mixed tumor (chondroid syringoma) of the scapula treated with staged margin-controlled excision. Am J Dermatopathol 2018;40(9):679–81.

38. Nguyen CM, Cassarino DS. Local recurrence of cutaneous mixed tumor (chondroid syringoma) as malignant mixed tumor of the thumb 20 years after initial diagnosis. J Cutan Pathol 2017;44(3):292–5.

39. Requena C, Brotons S, Sanmartín O, et al. Malignant chondroid syringoma of the face with bone invasion. Am J Dermatopathol 2013;35:395–8.

40. Won YY, Suh DW, Lew BL, et al. Syringoid eccrine carcinoma of the thigh. Ann Dermatol 2017;29(6):786–9.

41. Sidiropoulos M, Sade S, Al-Habeeb A, et al. Syringoid eccrine carcinoma: a clinicopathological and immunohistochemical study of four cases. J Clin Pathol 2011;64(9):788–92.

42. De Francesco V, Frattasio A, Pillon B, et al. Carcinosarcoma arising in a patient with multiple cylindromas. Am J Dermatopathol 2005;27(1):21–6.

43. Dai B, Kong YY, Cai X, et al. Spiradenocarcinoma, cylindrocarcinoma and spiradenocylindrocarcinoma: a clinicopathological study of nine cases. Histopathology 2014;65(5):658–66.

44. Staiger RD, Helmchen B, Papet C, et al. Spiradenocarcinoma: a comprehensive data review. Am J Dermatopathol 2017;39(10):715–25.

45. Beaulieu D, Fathi R, Mir A, et al. Spiradenocarcinoma treated with Mohs micrographic surgery. Dermatol Surg 2018. [Epub ahead of print].
46. Granter SR, Seeger K, Calonje E, et al. Malignant eccrine spiradenoma (spiradenocarcinoma): a clinicopathologic study of 12 cases. Am J Dermatopathol 2000; 22(2):97–103.
47. Brown CA, Lynch MC, Ueno CM. Mucinous adenocarcinoma of the scalp: primary cutaneous neoplasm versus underlying metastatic disease. Plast Reconstr Surg Glob Open 2018;6(4):e1761.
48. Kamalpour L, Brindise RT, Nodzenski M, et al. Primary cutaneous mucinous carcinoma: a systematic review and meta-analysis of outcomes after surgery. JAMA Dermatol 2014;150(4):380–4.
49. Miquelestorena-Standley E, Dujardin F, Arbion F. Recurrent primary cutaneous mucinous carcinoma with neuroendocrine differentiation: case report and review of the literature. J Cutan Pathol 2014;41(8):686–91.
50. Walker A, Mesinkovska NA, Emanuel PO, et al. Polymorphous sweat gland carcinoma: a report of two cases. J Cutan Pathol 2016;43(7):594–601.
51. Ronen S, Aguilera-Barrantes I, Giorgadze T, et al. Polymorphous sweat gland carcinoma: an immunohistochemical and molecular study. Am J Dermatopathol 2018;40(8):580–7.
52. Castanon MC, Casali SM, Lamim RF, et al. Microcystic adnexal carcinoma simulating scarring alopecia. An Bras Dermatol 2015;90(3 Suppl 1):36–8.
53. Gordon S, Fischer C, Martin A, et al. Microcystic adnexal carcinoma: a review of the literature. Dermatol Surg 2017;43(8):1012–6.
54. Llamas-Velasco M, Mentzel T, Rütten A. Primary cutaneous secretory carcinoma: a previously overlooked low-grade sweat gland carcinoma. J Cutan Pathol 2018; 45(3):240–5.
55. Droubi D, Zeitouni NC, Skitzki J, et al. Primary signet-ring cell carcinoma of the axilla. J Cutan Pathol 2013;40(2):269–73.
56. Misago N, Shinoda Y, Okawa T, et al. Histiocytoid and signet-ring cell carcinoma of the axilla: a type of cutaneous apocrine carcinoma equivalent to histiocytoid lobular carcinoma of the breast? Clin Exp Dermatol 2011;36(8):874–7.
57. Requena L, Prieto VG, Requena C, et al. Primary signet-ring cell/histiocytoid carcinoma of the eyelid: a clinicopathologic study of 5 cases and review of the literature. Am J Surg Pathol 2011;35(3):378–91.

Extramammary Paget's Disease

Mackenzie Asel, MD[a], Nicole R. LeBoeuf, MD, MPH[a,b],*

KEYWORDS

- Extramammary Paget's disease • EMPD • Diagnosis • Prognosis
- Management options

KEY POINTS

- Extramammary Paget's disease (EMPD) is a rare cutaneous malignancy that primarily affects the anogenital region in the elderly.
- EMPD may be associated with a contiguous or synchronous malignancy and evaluation, and follow-up monitoring for additional malignancies is warranted.
- There are no randomized controlled trials to guide management, but when possible without inducing severe morbidity or functional impairment, definitive surgical therapy is optimal, using Mohs surgery when available.

CLINICAL PRESENTATION

Extramammary Paget's disease (EMPD) most commonly presents in the sixth to eighth decades at anatomic sites rich in apocrine glands, especially the vulva, penis, scrotum, perineum, and perianal area. It has been less frequently reported in other sites, including axillae, umbilicus, eyelid, external auditory meatus, and ectopic locations on other parts of the head, trunk, and extremities. It is most common in Caucasians and in women, with the vulva being its location of predilection, but in Asian populations, there is a male predominance. It is a rare neoplasm; the exact incidence is unknown.

Classically, EMPD presents as a pink or red plaque with typical white "cake-icing" scaling or ulceration (**Fig. 1**A). These "strawberries and cream" plaques are often initially disregarded by patients or misdiagnosed by clinicians, leading to delays in treatment of up to many years. It may be mistaken for candidiasis or dermatophytosis, eczema, psoriasis, lichen sclerosus, contact dermatitis, cutaneous lymphoma,

Any relevant commercial or financial conflicts of interest: None; Any funding sources: None.
[a] Department of Dermatology, The Centers for Melanoma and Cutaneous Oncology, Dana-Farber Cancer Institute, 450 Brookline Avenue, Boston, MA 02115, USA; [b] Dana-Farber/Brigham and Women's Cancer Center, 450 Brookline Avenue, Boston, MA 02115, USA
* Corresponding author. The Center for Cutaneous Oncology, Dana-Farber/Brigham and Women's Cancer Center, 450 Brookline Avenue, Boston, MA 02115.
E-mail address: nleboeuf@bwh.harvard.edu

Hematol Oncol Clin N Am 33 (2019) 73–85
https://doi.org/10.1016/j.hoc.2018.09.003
0889-8588/19/© 2018 Elsevier Inc. All rights reserved.

hemonc.theclinics.com

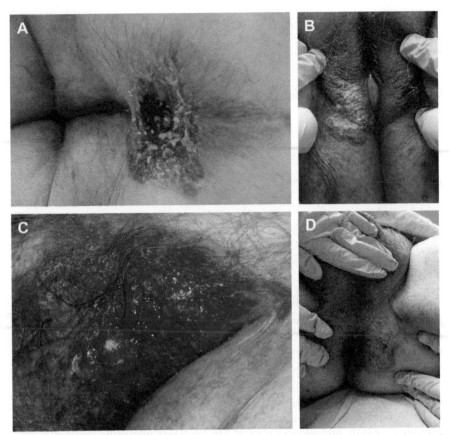

Fig. 1. (A) Perianal EMPD with white "cake-icing"–type scale. (B) EMPD of the vulva, with the classic "strawberries and cream" morphology showing a red plaque with distinct white scale. (C) Similar findings on the lateral scrotum extending beyond the inguinal fold and (D) on the medial buttock, extending into the perineum. Each case highlights the challenge of defining a clinical border in order to obtain a clear surgical margin.

melanoma, squamous cell carcinoma, and others, although on close inspection regardless of site of origin, its morphology is quite distinctive (**Fig. 1**B–D). Symptoms include pain, itching, burning, and weeping. Although topicals may provide temporary relief, EMPD does not resolve with topical anti-inflammatories or antifungals. As a general rule, it is prudent to biopsy any suspected chronic "dermatosis" of the ano-genital region that does not resolve with therapy in order to rule out this and other neoplasms.

PATHOGENESIS

The pathogenesis of primary EMPD is not well understood. Primary intraepidermal EMPD may arise from pluripotent cells in the epidermis and/or adnexae (possibly sweat glands or hair follicles). The condition may be derived from Toker cells, which are mammary gland–related cells found in the nipple and vulva. "Secondary" EMPD is generally accepted to be due to direct extension of an adjacent malignancy or in cases where an occult underlying malignancy is identified. The mechanism by which noncontiguous EMPD might develop is not understood.

DIAGNOSIS

The diagnosis of EMPD is established by skin biopsy, which reveals large cells with abundant amphophilic cytoplasm scattered with buckshot distribution or arranged in nests throughout all layers of epidermis; the tumor cells may crush the basal layer. The staining pattern is important to distinguish Paget's disease from other intraepidermal tumors with pagetoid spread. Paget's cells are usually positive for low-molecular-weight cytokeratins (including CK7, although this is nonspecific) and epithelial membrane antigen. Gross cystic disease fluid protein-15 is typically positive in primary EMPD and negative in secondary EMPD. Likewise, mucin core protein MUC5AC is frequently positive in primary EMPD and less often in secondary EMPD, and when primary EMPD becomes invasive, MUC5AC expression is often decreased or lost. CK20 is usually positive in secondary EMPD and negative in primary EMPD, but it is not specific. The use of immunohistochemical marker panels (including those previously mentioned as well as melanocytic markers, carcinoembryonic antigen [CEA], p63, and others) is important to rule out melanoma and squamous cell carcinoma in situ.[1] The staining pattern may also be helpful for prognostication purposes.[2]

WORKUP

In most patients, EMPD arises primarily in the skin, without a separate concomitant cancer. However, a minority of cases represents epidermotropic metastases of an associated sweat gland carcinoma or a distant malignancy, via contiguous spread or synchronous in diagnosis. These associated cancers may include carcinoma of the rectum, stomach, bladder, urethra, prostate, cervix, or breast. As such, a malignancy workup is recommended. The associated underlying malignancy rate ranges from 4% to 58% in the literature, with the wide variation likely related to heterogeneous time intervals and disparate interpretations about whether the reported malignancy is truly related to EMPD.

In all patients with EMPD, a thorough review of systems, full skin, breast, abdominal, pelvic, and lymph node examination should be followed by complete diagnostic testing; this extends beyond standard age-appropriate malignancy screenings. Although there is no standard approach to the required workup, studies suggested by Lam and Funaro,[3] in a comprehensive review from 2010 in addition to the above, include gynecologic evaluation (including colposcopy, Pap smear, and pelvic ultrasound), urologic evaluation (including cystoscopy with or without uroscan), colonoscopy, and, in the case of invasive EMPD, serum CEA. Many use advanced imaging, such as computed tomography or PET scan. An algorithm for cancer screening was more recently proposed, which calls for, in addition to history, examination and age-appropriate cancer screenings, and the following investigations: serial sectioning with staining to evaluate for invasive disease and underlying carcinoma, urine cytology and colonoscopy plus either prostate-specific antigen and digital rectal examination for men or Pap smear and mammography for women. The algorithm also recommends lymph node evaluation when invasive EMPD or contiguous invasive malignancy is present.[4] There are no guidelines about the frequency with which cancer screening should be repeated. Patients should certainly be followed closely over the long term, and clinicians should have a low index of suspicion to work up any new or unexplained signs or symptoms over time. The tissue's immunohistochemical staining pattern can shed some light on whether a case of EMPD is primary or secondary and, if secondary, heighten suspicion for the source of the metastasis.[5] Regardless of the staining pattern, however, a thorough search for the above associated malignancies is indicated with at least the minimum screening recommended. Interestingly, the role of cancer screening in patients with primary noninvasive EMPD of the vulva has recently been questioned, and further investigation is warranted across clinical sites.[6]

PROGNOSIS

Although primary EMPD is, by definition, not due to a systemic malignancy, invasive primary EMPD can be life threatening. In addition to EMPD's associated mortality, there are also severe implications for morbidity due to the disease and its treatment.

It is well established that individuals with invasive EMPD fare worse than those with in situ disease. Level of invasion is associated with nodal metastasis,[7,8] distant metastasis,[9] higher recurrence rate,[10] shorter mean time to recurrence,[11] decreased disease-specific survival,[11–15] and decreased overall survival.[16] Several studies use a threshold of 1-mm dermal invasion to stratify the degree of risk.[7,13,17] The 5-year disease-specific survival is 94.9% for patients with localized disease, 84.9% for those with regional disease, and 52.5% for those with distant disease. The mean disease-specific survival is 358.9 months, 248.5 months, and 136.3 months in each group, respectively.[18]

MANAGEMENT
Surgical Approaches

Historically, the standard approach to treatment of EMPD has been surgical excision. However, because of the tumor's multifocal nature, irregular shape, and indistinct boundaries, resection margins are frequently positive and local recurrences are common. Because surgery has also been the mainstay of treatment of local recurrences, patients can develop mutilating scarring and poor functional outcomes. When definitive clearance is possible, it should be considered first line after a discussion with the patient of the risks and benefits of alternative approaches.

Given the clinically indistinct margins, subclinical extension, high local recurrence rates, sensitive anatomic locations, and potential for metastasis, Mohs micrographic surgery is preferred. This tissue-sparing approach, when performed by a trained Mohs surgeon, allows for a greater likelihood of clearing operable tumors while leaving normal skin and mucosa intact; this is critical in areas with functionally important anatomic structures. Recurrence rates after Mohs remain higher for EMPD as compared with Mohs for other cutaneous malignancies, in part because of the irregular extensions of the tumor and in part because EMPD is more difficult to recognize microscopically. Despite its potential shortcomings, Mohs offers some advantages over standard excision. Rates of positive margin, which is associated with higher recurrence risk (hazard ratio 3.55, 95% confidence interval 1.74–7.24), with Mohs versus excision are reported to be 8% versus 22%,[19] 9% versus 44%,[20] 3.4% versus 33% for positive margin.[21] Rates of recurrence range from 8% to 26% for Mohs versus 33% to 60% for excision in published series.[22,23]

Although wide local excision has historically been the standard approach for treatment of EMPD, often leading to vulvectomy, emasculation surgery, and even abdominoperineal resection, much of the recent literature focuses on the use of Mohs and specific modifications to Mohs rather than conventional surgery for treatment of EMPD. There remain questions about whether margin status or margin width correlate with recurrence risk, making recommendations for wide excision difficult. One retrospective review of women with primary vulvar intraepithelial EMPD showed no correlation between disease recurrence and microscopic margin status ($P = .20$) among

28 patients over a median follow-up of 49 months (range 3–186 months).[24] In a retrospective review of men and women with EMPD, 28 patients underwent excision with a wide (>2 cm) margin, and 38 had a narrow (≤2 cm) margin. Local recurrence did not correlate with margin size (P = .155). Preoperative mapping biopsies were performed in 45 of these patients (68%), and use of mapping biopsy did not correlate with local recurrence (P = 1.000).[16]

There are many studies investigating the role (if any) of preoperative mapping biopsies, intraoperative frozen sections, and other techniques to maximize the efficacy of surgery, which may be particularly relevant when Mohs is not available.[25–31] Processing the peripheral and deep margin via Mohs, while sending the central portion for conventional pathology in order to assess tumor depth for prognostic purposes, is also reasonable.[26] Despite the lack of randomized controlled trials, there is a compelling body of knowledge to suggest that Mohs is preferable over wide excision for the treatment of EMPD.

Multiple studies have demonstrated a substantial risk of sentinel lymph node (SLN) metastasis in patients with primary invasive EMPD, with a reported incidence ranging from 16.9% to 37%, whereas SLN metastasis is absent in patients with in situ disease.[32–34] The rate of lymph node metastasis in patients without lymphadenopathy was 15% according to one study.[35] The prognostic significance of sentinel lymph node positivity is evident; lymph node metastasis is a predictor of overall survival, with one study reporting a 5-year survival rate of 100% in SLN-negative patients as compared with 24% in SLN-positive patients (P = .0001).[33] Despite this information, there is uncertainty surrounding patient selection for sentinel lymph node biopsy. Given the low morbidity associated with the procedure, as well as the fact that 30% of patients initially diagnosed with in situ disease on biopsy are subsequently found to have invasive disease, a low threshold for SLN biopsy may be reasonable.[32] It has been suggested that SLN biopsy is warranted in all patients with EMPD, except those whose primary tumor is definitely restricted to the epidermis on complete histologic evaluation.[8]

In the setting of a positive SLN, debate continues about whether completion lymphadenectomy is warranted. A few studies have attempted to answer this question. Tsutsumida and colleagues[36] suggested an algorithm in which individuals with clinical or pathologic lymph node metastasis undergo wide local excision plus therapeutic lymph node dissection. In the absence of clinical or pathologic lymph node metastasis, wide local excision only is performed, and if it reveals invasion to the reticular dermis or subcutis, then elective lymph node dissection follows. Their approach is based on the observation that the 5-year survival rate was 100% in patients with in situ or microinvasive disease but 33.3% in patients with invasion to the reticular dermis and 0% in patients with invasion in to the subcutis. Matsushita and colleagues,[37] on the other hand, suggest that the benefit of lymph node dissection depends on the size of the primary tumor and the tumor burden in affected lymph nodes. In the study on SLN biopsy previously mentioned, 6 of 10 patients with positive SLNs agreed to total lymphadenectomy; 4 of the 6 were free of disease over a follow-up period of 17 to 37 months. Two of the 4 patients who refused lymphadenectomy were alive with distant metastasis; one died of disease, and another died of a different disease.[32] Given the controversy, each patient's tumor, risk factors, and comorbidities must be considered in developing the treatment plan. As previously discussed, the above algorithms that involve wide excision with sentinel lymph node biopsy would preferentially be adjusted to Mohs surgery with coordinated sentinel lymph node biopsy based on available data.

Nonsurgical Approaches

Because of the inherent limitations of surgery for extirpating tumors with clinically ill-defined margins and subclinical extension, a nonsurgical approach to treatment offers an alluring strategy. More conservative treatments of EMPD are also emerging in efforts to decrease the morbidity associated with surgery, particularly given the high recurrence rates. However, there are limited data about the efficacy of these alternatives; as such, selection of a management plan requires cautious clinical judgment and a thorough discussion of risks, benefits, and alternatives with the patient.

Radiation therapy

A systematic review of literature regarding the use of radiation therapy for EMPD over the last 30 years was recently published.[38] All studies included more than one patient with histologically confirmed EMPD, treated with beam or surface conformal applicator brachytherapy. All were retrospective analyses. Collectively, 19 studies and 195 patients were encompassed. There was significant heterogeneity in radiation doses, fractionation, technique, and clinical settings. The use of definitive radiotherapy for primary or recurrent disease (not specifying depth) with doses of 30 to 80.2 Gy is associated with 50% to 100% complete response rates and local relapse or recurrence from 0% to 80% of cases. Postoperative adjuvant radiotherapy in doses 32 to 64.8 Gy resulted in local recurrence or persistence in 0% to 62.5%. In small studies of in situ EMPD, 40 Gy in 9 to 20 fractions resulted in complete response in 4 patients.[39] Radiation therapy was well tolerated across studies. Although large data sets show overall worse outcomes when radiotherapy is used for definitive disease, these are retrospective in nature and do not take into account tumor- and patient-specific factors, and conclusions cannot be drawn.[18,40] Given the extraordinary morbidity associated with surgery in many cases, as well as the patient population most commonly affected, radiation therapy should certainly be considered particularly when in situ disease is suspected, and surgery would result in severe disfigurement or functional impairment.

Additional skin directed therapies

Imiquimod is a topical immunomodulatory cream that acts as an agonist of toll-like receptor 7, thereby inducing innate and cell-mediated immune responses. It is approved for treatment of condyloma acuminata, actinic keratosis, superficial basal cell carcinoma, and, in immunocompromised patients, antiviral-resistant genital herpes simplex. It has been used for a variety of off-label indications and was first reported to treat 2 cases of EMPD in 2002.[41] Although there are no randomized trials, multiple observational studies since then have demonstrated the potential role of imiquimod in the treatment of EMPD. Treatment regimens generally use 2 or 3 times weekly application, and durations in the literature range from 2 to 54 weeks (mean 12.4 weeks). When used as primary treatment, complete response rates range from 52% to 75% and partial responses range from 16% to 28%.[42–47] Relapse rates appear to be high, and long-term follow-up or even persistent treatment may be warranted. Further prospective studies are underway. Given ease of application and low morbidity, its use should be considered on a case-by-case basis.

There remain many unanswered questions about the optimal use of imiquimod, including patient selection, frequency, and duration.[48,49] It is plausible, although uncertain whether different anatomic sites (such as mucosal vs cutaneous surfaces) respond with different efficacy to topical imiquimod. An added layer of complexity is to consider whether to use imiquimod as monotherapy versus adjuvant or neoadjuvant therapy. Indeed, imiquimod has been used successfully in combination with either photodynamic therapy or tazorotene.[50–52] It has been used as a way to debulk a tumor before surgery and as an attempt to prevent recurrence after surgery or radiation.[53,54]

Topical *5-fluorouracil* is a pyrimidine analogue that acts by inhibiting synthesis of DNA and RNA. Although it has a variety of uses for cutaneous neoplasms and is approved for treatment of actinic keratosis and superficial basal cell carcinoma, it does not appear to be effective in the treatment of EMPD.[55,56] A potential role for using fluorouracil to help delineate tumor margins before surgery has been suggested in separate case reports.[57,58] Although a neoadjuvant or adjuvant indication for fluoro-uracil may be conceivable, the level of evidence is weak, and so fluorouracil should not be relied on, given the availability of other modalities.

Bleomycin is sometimes found listed among the options for localized treatment of EMPD, but evidence for its use is extremely scant.[59] Similarly, *cryotherapy* has been reported in a handful of case reports but does not have sufficient evidence base for clinical use.[60–62] Topical *retinoids* have been used in combination with imiqui-mod, *photodynamic therapy (PDT)*, and topical fluorouracil, but data to support their use are lacking.[52,63,64]

With PDT, patients are exposed to a photosensitizing agent (topical aminolevulinic acid, methylaminolevulinate, or systemic porfimer sodium) and then exposed to visible light, which creates reactive oxygen species and results in selective destruction of neoplastic tissue. The advantages of PDT include cancer selectivity as well as the abil-ity to be repeated over time without additive risk (such as scarring). It is minimally inva-sive, treats both clinically and subclinically involved areas, and results in good cosmetic and functional outcomes. It may be more tolerable in elderly individuals who are poor surgical candidates. Response rates range from 66% to 78%.[65–69] Relapse rates are high, similar to other nonsurgical modalities. Patients have been shown to have improved symptoms and quality of life.[65,67] PDT has also been used in small studies in combination with surgery, resulting in lower recurrence rates and smaller wound size.[50,51,69]

Laser therapy is among the alternative treatment options for EMPD, but the level of evidence is weak. There are a few single case reports about the successful use of Nd:YAG laser or CO_2 laser alone or in combination with photodynamic diagnosis.[70–72] There are also a few observational studies in which laser is used in combination with surgery, photodynamic therapy, or both, so it is unclear to what extent laser contrib-utes to efficacy.[73–76] Other studies report a high recurrence rate after laser treat-ment.[77–79] Of note, ablation by carbon dioxide laser is a painful procedure, often involving a sensitive anatomic region when used for the treatment of EMPD.

Systemic therapy

For patients with advanced EMPD, several traditional chemotherapeutics have been used, including 5-fluorouracil, cisplatin, carboplatin, docetaxel, paclitaxel, irinotecan, epirubicin, vincristine, mitomycin C, and S-1. Recently, increasing attention has been directed to the role of human epidermal growth receptor 2 (HER-2) signaling in various malignancies and its therapeutic implications. Trastuzumab is a humanized mono-clonal antibody that selectively inhibits HER-2. It is approved for use in HER-2–over-expressing breast cancer and metastatic gastric cancer. Multiple studies have demonstrated HER-2 overexpression in lesions of EMPD.[80,81] In addition, some studies show a significant correlation between the presence of invasion and strong positivity for HER-2, and/or the presence of lymph node metastasis and strong HER-2 positivity.[82–84] There are reports in which trastuzumab (either alone or in combination with chemotherapy, such as paclitaxel or docetaxel/carboplatin, or in combination or sequence with targeted agents, such as pertuzumab, lapatinib, and ado-trastuzumab emtansine) has resulted in regression of primary tumors and, when present, their metastases.[85–91] Of course, although targeted therapies provide a potentially promising option for patients with unresectable, invasive, and/or metastatic disease, more data are needed about their optimal use in EMPD. There are currently no data on the use of systemic immunotherapy in metastatic EMPD. However, given responses to topical imiquimod, it is reasonable to consider. There are ongoing trials using intralesional and systemic immunotherapy that allow for inclusion of EMPD.

Despite all of the above data regarding the management of EMPD, there have been no randomized controlled trials to assess objectively.[92]

SUMMARY

In conclusion, EMPD is a rare but morphologically distinct cutaneous malignancy that predominately affects the anogenital region of elderly people. A critical component of its management is evaluation for an underlying malignancy, particularly of the genitourinary or gastrointestinal tract. There are many treatment options, but a paucity of data to guide best practice. If curative surgery is possible without significant morbidity and functional impairment, definitive removal with complete circumferential margin assessment, ideally via tissue-sparing Mohs surgery, should be used. Given the high recurrence rates across all other modalities, clinicians should consider the tumor's characteristics (location, invasion, and so forth) as well as the patient's overall health status and goals when deciding upon a management plan. Prospective trials are needed.

REFERENCES

1. Ivan D, Lazar A, Calonje E. Cutaneous metastases and Paget's disease of the skin. In: Calonje E, Brenn T, Lazar A, et al, editors. McKee's pathology of the skin: with clinical correlations. 4th edition. Saint Louis (MO): Elsevier/Saunders; 2012.
2. Cohen JM, Granter SR, Werchniak AE. Risk stratification in extramammary Paget disease. Clin Exp Dermatol 2015;40(5):473–8.
3. Lam C, Funaro D. Extramammary Paget's disease: summary of current knowledge. Dermatol Clin 2010;28(4):807–26.
4. Schmitt AR, Long BJ, Weaver AL, et al. Evidence-based screening recommendations for occult cancers in the setting of newly diagnosed extramammary paget disease. Mayo Clin Proc 2018;93(7):877–83.
5. Perrotto J, Abbott JJ, Ceilley RI, et al. The role of immunohistochemistry in discriminating primary from secondary extramammary Paget disease. Am J Dermatopathol 2010;32(2):137–43.
6. van der Linden M, Schuurman MS, Bulten J, et al. Stop routine screening for associated malignancies in cutaneous non-invasive vulvar Paget disease? Br J Dermatol 2018. [Epub ahead of print].
7. Shiomi T, Noguchi T, Nakayama H, et al. Clinicopathological study of invasive extramammary Paget's disease: subgroup comparison according to invasion depth. J Eur Acad Dermatol Venereol 2013;27(5):589–92.
8. Hatta N, Morita R, Yamada M, et al. Sentinel lymph node biopsy in patients with extramammary Paget's disease. Dermatol Surg 2004;30(10):1329–34.
9. Iacoponi S, Zalewski K, Fruscio R, et al. Prognostic factors for recurrence and survival among patients with invasive vulvar Paget disease included in the VULCAN study. Int J Gynaecol Obstet 2016;133(1):76–9.

10. Pierie JP, Choudry U, Muzikansky A, et al. Prognosis and management of extramammary Paget's disease and the association with secondary malignancies. J Am Coll Surg 2003;196(1):45–50.
11. Parker LP, Parker JR, Bodurka-Bevers D, et al. Paget's disease of the vulva: pathology, pattern of involvement, and prognosis. Gynecol Oncol 2000;77(1):183–9.
12. Dai B, Kong YY, Chang K, et al. Primary invasive carcinoma associated with penoscrotal extramammary Paget's disease: a clinicopathological analysis of 56 cases. BJU Int 2015;115(1):153–60.
13. Shu B, Shen XX, Chen P, et al. Primary invasive extramammary Paget disease on penoscrotum: a clinicopathological analysis of 41 cases. Hum Pathol 2016;47(1): 70–7.
14. Ito Y, Igawa S, Ohishi Y, et al. Prognostic indicators in 35 patients with extramammary Paget's disease. Dermatol Surg 2012;38(12):1938–44.
15. Ito T, Kaku Y, Nagae K, et al. Tumor thickness as a prognostic factor in extramammary Paget's disease. J Dermatol 2015;42(3):269–75.
16. Hatta N, Yamada M, Hirano T, et al. Extramammary Paget's disease: treatment, prognostic factors and outcome in 76 patients. Br J Dermatol 2008;158(2):313–8.
17. Crawford D, Nimmo M, Clement PB, et al. Prognostic factors in Paget's disease of the vulva: a study of 21 cases. Int J Gynecol Pathol 1999;18(4):351–9.
18. Karam A, Dorigo O. Treatment outcomes in a large cohort of patients with invasive Extramammary Paget's disease. Gynecol Oncol 2012;125(2):346–51.
19. O'Connor WJ, Lim KK, Zalla MJ, et al. Comparison of mohs micrographic surgery and wide excision for extramammary Paget's disease. Dermatol Surg 2003;29(7): 723–7.
20. Kim SJ, Thompson AK, Zubair AS, et al. Surgical treatment and outcomes of patients with extramammary Paget disease: a cohort study. Dermatol Surg 2017; 43(5):708–14.
21. Long B, Schmitt AR, Weaver AL, et al. A matter of margins: Surgical and pathologic risk factors for recurrence in extramammary Paget's disease. Gynecol Oncol 2017;147(2):358–63.
22. Hendi A, Brodland DG, Zitelli JA. Extramammary Paget's disease: surgical treatment with Mohs micrographic surgery. J Am Acad Dermatol 2004;51(5):767–73.
23. Bae JM, Choi YY, Kim H, et al. Mohs micrographic surgery for extramammary Paget disease: a pooled analysis of individual patient data. J Am Acad Dermatol 2013;68(4):632–7.
24. Black D, Tornos C, Soslow RA, et al. The outcomes of patients with positive margins after excision for intraepithelial Paget's disease of the vulva. Gynecol Oncol 2007;104(3):547–50.
25. Kaku-Ito Y, Ito T, Tsuji G, et al. Evaluation of mapping biopsies for extramammary Paget disease: a retrospective study. J Am Acad Dermatol 2018;78(6): 1171–7.e4.
26. O'Connor EA, Hettinger PC, Neuburg M, et al. Extramammary Paget's disease: a novel approach to treatment using a modification of peripheral Mohs micrographic surgery. Ann Plast Surg 2012;68(6):616–20.
27. Thomas CJ, Wood GC, Marks VJ. Mohs micrographic surgery in the treatment of rare aggressive cutaneous tumors: the Geisinger experience. Dermatol Surg 2007;33(3):333–9.
28. Kim BJ, Park SK, Chang H. The effectiveness of mapping biopsy in patients with extramammary paget's disease. Arch Plast Surg 2014;41(6):753–8.

29. Kato T, Fujimoto N, Fujii N, et al. Mapping biopsy with punch biopsies to determine surgical margin in extramammary Paget's disease. J Dermatol 2013; 40(12):968–72.
30. Shaco-Levy R, Bean SM, Vollmer RT, et al. Paget disease of the vulva: a histologic study of 56 cases correlating pathologic features and disease course. Int J Gynecol Pathol 2010;29(1):69–78.
31. Stacy D, Burrell MO, Franklin EW 3rd. Extramammary Paget's disease of the vulva and anus: use of intraoperative frozen-section margins. Am J Obstet Gynecol 1986;155(3):519–23.
32. Nakamura Y, Fujisawa Y, Ishikawa M, et al. Usefulness of sentinel lymph node biopsy for extramammary Paget disease. Br J Dermatol 2012;167(4):954–6.
33. Ogata D, Kiyohara Y, Yoshikawa S, et al. Usefulness of sentinel lymph node biopsy for prognostic prediction in extramammary Paget's disease. Eur J Dermatol 2016;26(3):254–9.
34. Kusatake K, Harada Y, Mizumoto K, et al. Usefulness of sentinel lymph node biopsy for the detection of metastasis in the early stage of extramammary Paget's disease. Eur J Dermatol 2015;25(2):156–61.
35. Fujisawa Y, Yoshino K, Kiyohara Y, et al. The role of sentinel lymph node biopsy in the management of invasive extramammary Paget's disease: multi-center, retrospective study of 151 patients. J Dermatol Sci 2015;79(1):38–42.
36. Tsutsumida A, Yamamoto Y, Minakawa H, et al. Indications for lymph node dissection in the treatment of extramammary Paget's disease. Dermatol Surg 2003;29(1):21–4.
37. Matsushita S, Hatanaka M, Katsue H, et al. Possible effectiveness of lymph node dissection in patients with extramammary Paget's disease. J Dermatol 2013; 40(7):574–5.
38. Tagliaferri L, Casa C, Macchia G, et al. The role of radiotherapy in extramammary paget disease: a systematic review. Int J Gynecol Cancer 2018;28(4):829–39.
39. Cai Y, Sheng W, Xiang L, et al. Primary extramammary Paget's disease of the vulva: the clinicopathological features and treatment outcomes in a series of 43 patients. Gynecol Oncol 2013;129(2):412–6.
40. Yao H, Xie M, Fu S, et al. Survival analysis of patients with invasive extramammary Paget disease: implications of anatomic sites. BMC Cancer 2018;18(1):403.
41. Zampogna JC, Flowers FP, Roth WI, et al. Treatment of primary limited cutaneous extramammary Paget's disease with topical imiquimod monotherapy: two case reports. J Am Acad Dermatol 2002;47(4 Suppl):S229–35.
42. Luyten A, Sorgel P, Clad A, et al. Treatment of extramammary Paget disease of the vulva with imiquimod: a retrospective, multicenter study by the German Colposcopy Network. J Am Acad Dermatol 2014;70(4):644–50.
43. Dogan A, Hilal Z, Krentel H, et al. Paget's disease of the vulva treated with imiquimod: case report and systematic review of the literature. Gynecol Obstet Invest 2017;82(1):1–7.
44. Knight SR, Proby C, Ziyaie D, et al. Extramammary Paget disease of the perianal region: the potential role of imiquimod in achieving disease control. J Surg Case Rep 2016;2016(8) [pii:rjw110].
45. Cowan RA, Black DR, Hoang LN, et al. A pilot study of topical imiquimod therapy for the treatment of recurrent extramammary Paget's disease. Gynecol Oncol 2016;142(1):139–43.
46. Sawada M, Kato J, Yamashita T, et al. Imiquimod 5% cream as a therapeutic option for extramammary Paget's disease. J Dermatol 2018;45(2):216–9.

47. van der Linden M, Meeuwis K, van Hees C, et al. The paget trial: a multicenter, observational cohort intervention study for the clinical efficacy, safety, and immunological response of topical 5% imiquimod cream for vulvar paget disease. JMIR Res Protoc 2017;6(9):e178.

48. Jim On SC, Izumi AK. Extramammary Paget disease: failure to respond to topical imiquimod 5%. J Am Acad Dermatol 2011;65(3):656–7.

49. Green JS, Burkemper NM, Fosko SW. Failure of extensive extramammary Paget disease of the inguinal area to clear with imiquimod cream, 5%: possible progression to invasive disease during therapy. Arch Dermatol 2011;147(6):704–8.

50. Jing W, Juan X, Li X, et al. Complete remission of two patients with recurrent and wide spread extramammary Paget disease obtained from 5-aminolevulinic acid-based photodynamic therapy and imiquimod combination treatment. Photodiagnosis Photodyn Ther 2014;11(3):434–40.

51. Apalla Z, Lallas A, Tsorova A, et al. Complete response of extramammary Paget's disease with imiquimod and PDT: Report of two cases. Photodermatol Photoimmunol Photomed 2018. [Epub ahead of print].

52. Frances L, Pascual JC, Leiva-Salinas M, et al. Extramammary Paget disease successfully treated with topical imiquimod 5% and tazarotene. Dermatol Ther 2014; 27(1):19–20.

53. Toledo F, Silvestre JF, Cuesta L, et al. Sequential use with imiquimod and surgery in extramammary Paget's disease. Dermatol Ther 2012;25(1):82–5.

54. Choi JH, Jue MS, Kim EJ, et al. Extramammary paget disease: minimal surgical therapy. Ann Dermatol 2013;25(2):213–7.

55. Haberman HF, Goodall J, Llewellyn M. Extramammary Paget's disease. Can Med Assoc J 1978;118(2):161–2.

56. Del Castillo LF, Garcia C, Schoendorff C, et al. Spontaneous apparent clinical resolution with histologic persistence of a case of extramammary Paget's disease: response to topical 5-fluorouracil. Cutis 2000;65(5):331–3.

57. Bewley AP, Bracka A, Staughton RC, et al. Extramammary Paget's disease of the scrotum: treatment with topical 5-fluorouracil and plastic surgery. Br J Dermatol 1994;131(3):445–6.

58. Eliezri YD, Silvers DN, Horan DB. Role of preoperative topical 5-fluorouracil in preparation for Mohs micrographic surgery of extramammary Paget's disease. J Am Acad Dermatol 1987;17(3):497–505.

59. Watring WG, Roberts JA, Lagasse LD, et al. Treatment of recurrent Paget's disease of the vulva with topical bleomycin. Cancer 1978;41(1):10–1.

60. Boulard C, Duval Modeste AB, Boullie MC, et al. Cryosurgery and photodynamic therapy for the treatment of Paget's disease of the vulva: two cases. Ann Dermatol Venereol 2013;140(4):282–6 [in French].

61. Neumann R. Extramammary Paget's disease associated with stomach cancer. Hautarzt 1986;37(10):568–70 [in German].

62. Gibson JR, Pequm JS, Baker H, et al. Multifocal extramammary Paget's disease. J R Soc Med 1983;76(5):426–7.

63. Magnano M, Loi C, Bardazzi F, et al. Methyl - aminolevulinic acid photodynamic therapy and topical tretinoin in a patient with vulvar extramammary Paget's disease. Dermatol Ther 2013;26(2):170–2.

64. Ye JN, Rhew DC, Yip F, et al. Extramammary Paget's disease resistant to surgery and imiquimod monotherapy but responsive to imiquimod combination topical chemotherapy with 5-fluorouracil and retinoic acid: a case report. Cutis 2006; 77(4):245–50.

65. Clement E, Sparsa A, Doffoel-Hantz V, et al. Photodynamic therapy for the treatment of extramammary Paget's disease. Ann Dermatol Venereol 2012;139(2): 103–8 [in French].
66. Nardelli AA, Stafinski T, Menon D. Effectiveness of photodynamic therapy for mammary and extra-mammary Paget's disease: a state of the science review. BMC Dermatol 2011;11:13.
67. Fontanelli R, Papadia A, Martinelli F, et al. Photodynamic therapy with M-ALA as non surgical treatment option in patients with primary extramammary Paget's disease. Gynecol Oncol 2013;130(1):90–4.
68. Al Yousef A, Boccara O, Moyal-Barracco M, et al. Incomplete efficacy of 5-amino-levulinic acid (5 ALA) photodynamic therapy in the treatment of widespread extramammary Paget's disease. Photodermatol Photoimmunol Photomed 2012; 28(1):53–5.
69. Wang HW, Lv T, Zhang LL, et al. A prospective pilot study to evaluate combined topical photodynamic therapy and surgery for extramammary paget's disease. Lasers Surg Med 2013;45(5):296–301.
70. Weese D, Murphy J, Zimmern PE. Nd: YAG laser treatment of extramammary Paget's disease of the penis and scrotum. J Urol (Paris) 1993;99(5):269–71.
71. Valentine BH, Arena B, Green E. Laser ablation of recurrent Paget's disease of vulva and perineum. J Gynecol Surg 1992;8(1):21–4.
72. Becker-Wegerich PM, Fritsch C, Schulte KW, et al. Carbon dioxide laser treatment of extramammary Paget's disease guided by photodynamic diagnosis. Br J Dermatol 1998;138(1):169–72.
73. Zollo JD, Zeitouni NC. The Roswell Park Cancer Institute experience with extramammary Paget's disease. Br J Dermatol 2000;142(1):59–65.
74. Fukui T, Watanabe D, Tamada Y, et al. Photodynamic therapy following carbon dioxide laser enhances efficacy in the treatment of extramammary Paget's disease. Acta Derm Venereol 2009;89(2):150–4.
75. Bergen S, DiSaia PJ, Liao SY, et al. Conservative management of extramammary Paget's disease of the vulva. Gynecol Oncol 1989;33(2):151–6.
76. Ewing TL. Paget's disease of the vulva treated by combined surgery and laser. Gynecol Oncol 1991;43(2):137–40.
77. Louis-Sylvestre C, Haddad B, Paniel BJ. Paget's disease of the vulva: results of different conservative treatments. Eur J Obstet Gynecol Reprod Biol 2001; 99(2):253–5.
78. Lai YL, Yang WG, Tsay PK, et al. Penoscrotal extramammary Paget's disease: a review of 33 cases in a 20-year experience. Plast Reconstr Surg 2003;112(4): 1017–23.
79. Choi JB, Yoon ES, Yoon DK, et al. Failure of carbon dioxide laser treatment in three patients with penoscrotal extramammary Paget's disease. BJU Int 2001; 88(3):297–8.
80. Ogawa T, Nagashima Y, Wada H, et al. Extramammary Paget's disease: analysis of growth signal pathway from the human epidermal growth factor receptor 2 protein. Hum Pathol 2005;36(12):1273–80.
81. Brummer O, Stegner HE, Bohmer G, et al. HER-2/neu expression in Paget disease of the vulva and the female breast. Gynecol Oncol 2004;95(2):336–40.
82. Masuguchi S, Jinnin M, Fukushima S, et al. The expression of HER-2 in extramammary Paget's disease. Biosci Trends 2011;5(4):151–5.
83. Richter CE, Hui P, Buza N, et al. HER-2/NEU overexpression in vulvar Paget disease: the Yale experience. J Clin Pathol 2010;63(6):544–7.

84. Tanaka R, Sasajima Y, Tsuda H, et al. Human epidermal growth factor receptor 2 protein overexpression and gene amplification in extramammary Paget disease. Br J Dermatol 2013;168(6):1259–66.
85. Hanawa F, Inozume T, Harada K, et al. A case of metastatic extramammary Paget's disease responding to trastuzumab plus paclitaxel combination therapy. Case Rep Dermatol 2011;3(3):223–7.
86. Karam A, Berek JS, Stenson A, et al. HER-2/neu targeting for recurrent vulvar Paget's disease A case report and literature review. Gynecol Oncol 2008;111(3): 568–71.
87. Shin DS, Sherry T, Kallen ME, et al. Human epidermal growth factor receptor 2 (HER-2/neu)-directed therapy for rare metastatic epithelial tumors with HER-2 amplification. Case Rep Oncol 2016;9(2):298–304.
88. Barth P, Dulaimi Al-Saleem E, Edwards KW, et al. Metastatic extramammary Paget's disease of scrotum responds completely to single agent trastuzumab in a hemodialysis patient: case report, molecular profiling and brief review of the literature. Case Rep Oncol Med 2015;2015:895151.
89. Takahagi S, Noda H, Kamegashira A, et al. Metastatic extramammary Paget's disease treated with paclitaxel and trastuzumab combination chemotherapy. J Dermatol 2009;36(8):457–61.
90. Zhang X, Jin W, Zhu H, et al. Extramammary paget's disease in two brothers. Indian J Dermatol 2015;60(4):423.
91. Watanabe S, Takeda M, Takahama T, et al. Successful human epidermal growth receptor 2-targeted therapy beyond disease progression for extramammary Paget's disease. Invest New Drugs 2016;34(3):394–6.
92. Edey KA, Allan E, Murdoch JB, et al. Interventions for the treatment of Paget's disease of the vulva. Cochrane Database Syst Rev 2013;(10):CD009245.

Cutaneous Sarcomas

Mehul D. Bhatt, MD, MBA[a], Vinod E. Nambudiri, MD, MBA[b,c],*

KEYWORDS

- Cutaneous sarcomas • Kaposi sarcoma • Angiosarcoma
- Dermatofibrosarcoma protuberans • Cutaneous leiomyosarcoma
- Cutaneous oncology

KEY POINTS

- Cutaneous sarcomas are uncommon neoplasms arising from the skin and should be considered in the differential diagnosis of new or growing skin lesions. Cutaneous sarcomas often have an aggressive clinical course relative to other cutaneous malignancies.
- Kaposi sarcoma arises from cells of endothelial origin and may be classified into classic, endemic, acquired immunodeficiency syndrome–associated, or immunosuppression-related types. The histologic spectrum of disease is also variable.
- Angiosarcoma is a rare but typically aggressive cutaneous sarcoma that often presents as a bruiselike lesion. First-line treatment is combined surgical excision and radiation.

INTRODUCTION

Cutaneous sarcomas are rare malignancies that may present with a variety of clinical manifestations, may be associated with significant cutaneous and systemic burdens, and may have dramatic impacts on quality of life (**Box 1**). This article reviews clinical, diagnostic, and therapeutic aspects of 4 cutaneous sarcomas: Kaposi sarcoma (KS), cutaneous angiosarcoma, dermatofibrosarcoma protuberans, and cutaneous leiomyosarcoma.

KAPOSI SARCOMA
Epidemiology and Pathophysiology

KS, a cutaneous and systemic malignancy arising from aberrant proliferation of vascular and lymphatic tissues, was first characterized by the Hungarian

Disclosure: The authors have no relationships with any commercial company that has a direct financial interest in subject matter or materials discussed in this article or with a company making a competing product.
[a] Department of Dermatology, University of Pennsylvania, 3400 Civic Center Boulevard, Philadelphia, PA 19104, USA; [b] Department of Dermatology, Brigham and Women's Hospital, 221 Longwood Avenue, Boston, MA 02115, USA; [c] Cutaneous Oncology Program, Dana Farber Cancer Institute, Boston, MA 02215, USA
* Corresponding author. Department of Dermatology, Brigham and Women's Hospital, 221 Longwood Avenue, Boston, MA 02115.
E-mail address: vnambudiri@bwh.harvard.edu

Hematol Oncol Clin N Am 33 (2019) 87–101
https://doi.org/10.1016/j.hoc.2018.08.007
0889-8588/19/© 2018 Elsevier Inc. All rights reserved.

Box 1
Selected cutaneous sarcomas
Angiosarcoma
Kaposi Sarcoma
Dermatofibrosarcoma protuberans
Leiomyosarcoma
Atypical fibroxanthoma
Undifferentiated pleomorphic sarcoma
Epithelioid sarcoma
Clear cell sarcoma
Liposarcoma
Malignant fibrous histiocytoma
Fibromyxoid sarcoma
Angiomyxoma

dermatologist Moritz Kaposi in 1872.[1] The skin remains the most common site of involvement and disease presentation.

Since the initial characterization of KS, its etiopathogenesis has been linked to the human herpesvirus 8 (HHV8), also termed Kaposi sarcoma herpesvirus (KSHV). Four distinct clinical subtypes of KS are typically recognized: classic, acquired immunodeficiency syndrome (AIDS)–associated, endemic, and iatrogenic/immunosuppressed KS.

The epidemiology of KS varies worldwide by subtype. Classic KS typically occurs in individuals of Mediterranean or European Jewish descent. In the United States, classic KS is most commonly diagnosed in men (7:1 male/female predominance) with a mean age 74 years.[2] AIDS-associated KS prevalence corresponds with human immunodeficiency virus (HIV) prevalence globally; it is the most common neoplasm diagnosed in sub-Saharan Africa. In the United States, since the introduction of highly active antiretroviral therapy, the incidence of AIDS-associated KS has decreased steadily.[3] The overall United States incidence has decreased since 2000, although geographic and racial disparities in incidence and survival exist.[4]

The pathophysiologic linkage of KS to KSHV explained its increased prevalence among individuals with AIDS or iatrogenic immunosuppression. KSHV is necessary, but not sufficient, for development of KS lesions; the prevalence of HHV8 viremia is estimated to be as high as 30% across randomly screened populations,[5] vastly exceeding KS's prevalence. In individuals with KS, multiple molecular mechanisms contribute to malignancy development, including upregulation of specific oncogenes and growth factors leading to neoplastic differentiation and disruption of the surrounding vascular and inflammatory milieu.[6]

Clinical Features and Diagnosis

Classic KS is typically diagnosed in elderly Mediterranean, European, or Middle Eastern men. The lower extremities are most commonly involved.[2] Lesions initially develop as purpuric, violaceous macules or patches (**Fig. 1**), evolving into thicker papules, plaques, or larger nodules (**Fig. 2**). Lesions may be single or multiple at onset, and may be asymptomatic or present with pain, itch, bleeding, or other localized symptoms.

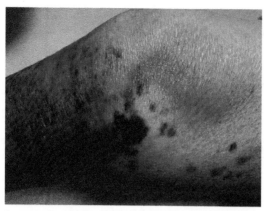

Fig. 1. Purpuric lesions on the thigh of patch-stage KS. Older tan-brown lesions are also visible.

When arising in association with HIV, KS typically develops in individuals with CD4 cell counts less than 200 cells/μL (although it may exceed this threshold); KS is considered an AIDS-defining illness. In addition to the lower extremities, the face and mucosal surfaces are common sites for AIDS-associated KS. With enhanced antiretroviral therapies available, the burden of AIDS-defining cancers should decrease in coming decades.[7] However, KS may arise during the immune reconstitution inflammatory syndrome following initiation of antiretroviral therapy for HIV, pointing to the role of inflammation in its pathogenesis.[8]

Endemic KS is native to the African continent and was identified before the HIV epidemic as a primarily pediatric malignancy.[9] In addition to onset at a younger age, patients typically present with marked lymphedema and lymphadenopathy in addition to cutaneous nodules. Endemic KS may also take on a fulminant, aggressive clinical presentation.

Iatrogenic KS arises in individuals on chronic immunosuppression (eg, solid organ transplant recipients or for autoimmune disorders). Incidence rates of KS in organ transplant recipients is more than 60-fold higher than in the general population.[10,11] Patients with immunosuppression-associated KS typically present at younger ages than those with classic KS, averaging 1 to 2 years posttransplant.[12]

Given its multifaceted cutaneous appearances (neoplastic and nonneoplastic differential diagnoses are presented in **Table 1**), tissue biopsy is necessary for making a definitive diagnosis of KS. Like the multiple clinical variants, KS shows a wide spectrum of histopathologic findings.[13] Characteristic findings include the presence of

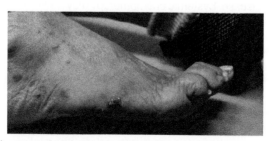

Fig. 2. Red to violaceous raised lesion on the medial foot of nodular KS. Smaller scattered early purpuric papular lesions are noted proximally.

Table 1	
Clinical differential diagnoses of cutaneous Kaposi sarcoma	
Benign vascular proliferations	Hemangioma, lymphangioma, pyogenic granuloma, arteriovenous malformations, atypical postradiation vascular proliferations
Benign vascular eruptions	Purpura, ecchymosis, hematoma, vasculitis, bacillary angiomatosis
Benign nonvascular proliferations	Dermatofibroma, keloid, hypertrophic scar
Benign pigmented lesions	Typical melanocytic nevi, dysplastic nevi
Malignant lesions	Melanoma, angiosarcoma, basal cell carcinoma, squamous cell carcinoma, Merkel cell carcinoma, cutaneous T-cell lymphoma, cutaneous B-cell lymphoma, cutaneous metastatic disease

spindle-shaped cells creating fine, slitlike dermal vascular spaces that displace normal, regularly oriented collagen. These spindled cells exhibit expression of KSHV on immunohistochemistry. As thicker plaques and nodules evolve, dermal vascular proliferation and inflammation typically progress. Variable features among different KS histopathologic subtypes (**Table 2**) include epidermal changes, cellular pleomorphisms, and edema.[13]

Treatment

Once a tissue diagnosis of KS is rendered, a thorough history and physical should be performed with particular attention to known risk factors (including HIV and immunosuppression) and areas of involvement beyond the skin (such as the oral/gastrointestinal mucosa). Appropriate screening of patients for HIV or for systemic involvement (eg, chest computed tomography [CT] for hemoptysis; fecal occult blood screening for gastrointestinal symptoms) should follow. For patients with HIV, viral load and antiviral treatment regimens should be determined.

For localized cutaneous disease, management varies based on disease extent. First and foremost, for patients with HIV-associated or immunosuppression-related KS, consideration must be given to systemic medication initiation (eg, antiretroviral therapy) or adjustment (eg, decreasing/switching immunosuppressive therapy). For a single cutaneous KS lesion, treatments may include surgery, radiation therapy, or intralesional or topical chemotherapy (**Table 3**). Local excision has varying rates of success but may be appropriate for management of single lesions. Radiation therapy most commonly involves localized fractionated external beam radiation therapy.[14,15] Intralesional chemotherapy, most commonly vinblastine, can also be used. Field radiation treatment or topical treatments (imiquimod or alitretinoin) may be used for widespread cutaneous disease. Systemic chemotherapy may also be considered for select patients, particularly under clinical trials.

Close observation and follow-up are hallmarks of KS management. Consensus recommendations regarding patients with AIDS-associated KS include evaluation every 3 months for the first year after diagnosis, and regular visits every 4 to 6 months in year 2 and every 6 months thereafter.[16]

CUTANEOUS ANGIOSARCOMA
Epidemiology and Pathophysiology

Cutaneous angiosarcoma (AS) arises from blood or lymphatic vessels, accounting for 1% of soft tissue sarcomas. Given the rarity of cutaneous AS, epidemiologic data

Table 2	
Histologic subtypes of Kaposi sarcoma and their typical features	
Patch-stage KS	• Earliest lesions • Subtle formation of vascular spaces
Plaque-stage KS	• Diffuse dermal vascular infiltrate • Haphazard fascicles create sievelike appearance
Nodular-stage KS	• Well-circumscribed proliferation of vascular neoplastic cells • Hyaline globules typically present • Ulceration may be present
Anaplastic (pleomorphic) KS	• Greater degree of nuclear and cellular pleomorphism than typical KS • Increased mitotic index • May be confused with other spindled neoplasms
Lymphedematous KS	• Ectatic lymphatic spaces or bullous spaces seen
Lymphangiomalike KS	• Interanastamosing vascular channels mimicking lymphangioma microscopically • Prominent promontory sign within vascular channels
Bullous KS	• Clinically bullous lesions, often in setting of endemic KS, with evidence of pronounced dermal or epidermal edema
Telangiectatic KS	• Presence of intensely congested ectatic vascular spaces, typically in nodular lesions
Hyperkeratotic (verrucous) KS	• Epidermal acanthosis and fibrosis overlying fibrotic epidermis
Keloidal KS	• Expanded dermis with dense keloidal collagen
Micronodular KS	• Small unencapsulated spindled proliferations within the dermis
Pyogenic granuloma–like KS	• Small lesions with peripheral epidermal collarette of scale mimicking pyogenic granuloma
Ecchymotic KS	• Extensive dermal red blood cell extravasation
Intravascular KS	• Intravascular spindled cell proliferations
Regressing KS	• Densely sclerotic stroma • Perivascular inflammatory infiltrate composed of plasma cells

Data from Grayson W, Pantanowitz L. Histological variants of cutaneous Kaposi sarcoma. Diagn Pathol 2008;3:31.

Table 3	
Selected treatments for cutaneous Kaposi sarcoma	
Topical Treatments	Imiquimod • 5% cream topically TIW Alitretinoin • 0.1% gel topically TID
Surgical Treatments	Wide local excision • Achievement of clear surgical margin
Radiation Treatment	External beam radiation therapy • 24 Gy in 12 fractions • 20 Gy in 5 fractions
Intralesional Chemotherapy	Vinblastine • 0.1 mL of 0.2 mg/mL solution injection
Systemic Chemotherapy	Liposomal doxorubicin • 20 mg/m^3 IV every 3 wk Paclitaxel • 100 mg/m^2 IV every 2 wk

Abbreviations: IV, intravenously; TID, 3 times a day; TIW, 3 times a week.

remain sparse.[17] In one large series of cutaneous AS, average age of diagnosis was 73 years, with a slight male predominance, and almost all occurred in white patients, who had higher incidence rates than African Americans.[17] The most common cutaneous AS sites are the head and neck, particularly the scalp. A pathophysiologic relationship to ultraviolet light may contribute to this distribution; AS incidences are higher among individuals with genetic susceptibility to ultraviolet-induced DNA damage.[18]

Additional risk factors for cutaneous AS include prior radiation exposure and chronic lymphedema. Radiation-induced AS frequently arises in areas previously treated for solid tumor malignancies (most often breast cancer).[17] The median time between radiation exposure and AS development is approximately 6 years.[19,20] Chronic lymphedema-associated AS (Stewart-Treves syndrome) arises secondary to lymphedema following postsurgical changes, hereditary disorders, chronic obesity, vascular overgrowth syndromes, or infectious diseases.

ASs are tumors arising from endothelial cells with either vascular or lymphatic features. Although the exact molecular pathogenesis remains to be elucidated, studies of vascular endothelial growth factor (VEGF) expression have consistently shown upregulation in multiple variants of AS, and additional genes involved in angiogenesis have also been identified as frequently mutated in AS.[21] For radiation-associated AS, amplification and overexpression of MYC, a family of transcription factors driving cell proliferation, has been observed.[22]

Diagnosis

Cutaneous AS typically occurs as a violaceous plaque arising on the head and neck or in a field of prior irradiation or chronic lymphedema; the initial appearance may mimic a persistent bruise. The aggressive nature of cutaneous AS can lead to rapid growth, ulceration, or invasion into adjacent structures. Given the highly vascular nature of AS, localized hemorrhage is common. With time, plaques may evolve into nodules or multicentric lesions. The pathologic extent of the tumor may exceed clinically visible borders, leading to frequently positive resection margins.

The hallmark histopathologic features of cutaneous AS include bizarre-appearing endothelial cells creating irregular, disarrayed vascular channels or sinusoids within the dermis, displacing normal, regularly oriented collagen. In less well-differentiated lesions, increasing cytologic disarray is observed. Similar to KS, multiple pathologic variants of AS have been identified (**Table 4**).[23] Consistent with the aggressive growth seen clinically, expansion of neoplastic vascular channels into subcutaneous fat and deeper structures often occurs.[24] Immunohistochemical expression of CD31, CD34, D2-40, and VEGFR3 can be seen, providing helpful distinction from nonendothelial neoplasms.[23] MYC expression can be seen in radiation-associated or other secondary forms of AS.[22]

Treatment

Treatment of cutaneous AS must account for its aggressive clinical course. Five-year survival after AS is approximately 50%, with lowest survival rates among individuals with head and neck lesions.[17] Surgery, radiation therapy, and systemic chemotherapy may be considered for cutaneous AS. Data point to improved outcomes, both overall and disease-specific survival, for patients treated with multimodal strategies (eg, excision plus radiation treatment).[25] Wide local excision (WLE) with clear margins should be sought, because positive margins predict worse outcomes. Similarly, tumors larger 5 cm are associated with worse outcomes.

The management of large cutaneous AS (ie, not amenable to excision) is an area of ongoing investigation. Multicenter retrospective analyses suggest multimodal

Table 4
Histologic subtypes of cutaneous angiosarcoma and their typical features

Well-differentiated Angiosarcoma	• Irregular anastomosis vascular channels with pleomorphic endothelial cells
Poorly Differentiated Angiosarcoma	• Ill-defined vascular structures, highly mitotically active pleomorphic endothelial cells • May show intracytoplasmic vacuoles or focal hemorrhage
Epithelioid Angiosarcoma	• Round epithelial cells with eosinophilic cytoplasm, vesicular nuclei

Rare Variants of Angiosarcoma
• Clear Cell Angiosarcoma
• Foam Cell Angiosarcoma
• Signet Ring Angiosarcoma
• Granular Cell Angiosarcoma
• Verrucous Angiosarcoma

treatment with systemic taxane-based chemotherapy plus radiation is particularly beneficial for large cutaneous AS.[26] Emerging studies of systemic agents for cutaneous AS have included pazopanib, bevacizumab, trabectedin, propranolol, and eribulin mesylate.[27] Interest has also emerged regarding immunotherapies (eg, pembrolizumab) in treating cutaneous AS.[28]

DERMATOFIBROSARCOMA PROTUBERANS

Dermatofibrosarcoma protuberans (DFSP) is a rare cutaneous soft tissue sarcoma with high potential for local invasion and recurrence, but rarely metastasizes. Histologic assessment is required for diagnosis, and surgical management with clear margins is the treatment of choice; improper removal accounts for high recurrence.[29] As DFSP's molecular pathogenesis has been elucidated, tyrosine kinase inhibitors have been used in unresectable or metastatic cases.[30]

Epidemiology

DFSP is rare, with 0.8 to 4.2 cases per million annually in the United States, accounting for 18% of cutaneous sarcomas.[31,32] DFSP most commonly arises in the third to fifth decades of life, and higher incidences are seen in men and African Americans.[32–34]

Pathogenesis

Greater than 90% of DFSP show chromosomal translocation t(17;22) resulting in the formation of collagen type I alpha I (COL1A1) and platelet-derived growth factor (PDGF) beta fusion gene. This fusion gene drives excessive PDGF receptor (a tyrosine kinase) activity, contributes to tumorigenesis, and is the rationale for targeted molecular therapy with tyrosine kinase inhibitors.[30,35–37]

Clinical Features and Histology

DFSP is an asymptomatic, slow-growing tumor initially manifesting as a skin-colored indurated plaque (**Fig. 3**). Over months to years, DFSP enlarges, becoming firm and nodular, and may exhibit ulceration, bleeding, or pain.[29,38] The risk of adherence to deeper structures (eg, fascia and bone) increases with tumor size.[39] The most common site for DFSP is on the trunk and proximal extremities.[32]

On histology, DFSP shows dermal spindle cell proliferations infiltrating subcutaneous fat creating a honeycomb appearance.[38] The tumor can invade tissue at a considerable distance from the central tumor.[29,40] Immunohistochemically, DFSP stains positively for CD34, hyaluronate, and vimentin, and negatively for factor XIIIa.[41] Histologic DFSP variants include Bednar, myxoid, giant cell fibroblastoma, sclerosing, atrophic, and fibrosarcomatous (**Table 5**).[39,42–46] The fibrosarcomatous variant exhibits higher rates of metastasis (14%) and poorer prognosis versus classic DFSP.[42–44,47] Classic DFSP exhibits metastatic rates of 1% to 4%, most commonly to the lungs.[48–50]

Diagnosis

Incisional or excisional biopsy is recommended for diagnosing DFSP, because fine-needle aspiration or superficial biopsy rarely provide enough tissue for accurate assessment.[51] After confirming diagnosis, a complete history and physical examination are warranted. If extensive extracutaneous extension is suspected, MRI can help define disease extent, and pulmonary evaluation with radiographs or CT may be warranted for chronic or large lesions.[52]

Treatment

For primary DFSP, surgical excision is the mainstay of treatment. Given its widely infiltrative nature, obtaining clear histologic margins is crucial for preventing recurrence and is the most important prognostic factor. Thorough peripheral and deep margin assessment, including deep fascia excision, is recommended.[51,52]

WLE or Mohs micrographic surgery (MMS) can be performed to obtain tumor clearance. Pooled data show local DFSP recurrence rate of 7.3% after WLE.[39] Although the overall rate is low, surgical margins ranged from less than 1 cm to 5 cm.[39,49,53] Current National Comprehensive Cancer Network (NCCN) guidelines recommend surgical margins of 2 to 4 cm.[51] If WLE is performed, closure may be delayed until final margins are cleared histologically.[54]

MMS offers immediate microscopic examination of all margins at excision. Primary DFSP recurrence rates after MMS are approximately 1%; systematic review shows

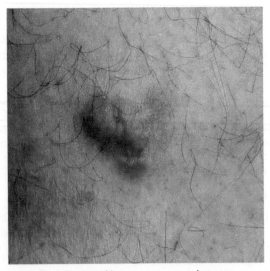

Fig. 3. Clinical appearance of dermatofibrosarcoma protuberans.

Table 5
Histologic subtypes of Dermatofibrosarcoma Protuberans and their typical features

Histologic Variant	Characteristics and Features
Bednar	• Pigmented variant: melanin-containing dendritic cells mixed among spindle cells • Represents 1% of all cases of DFSP
Myxoid	• Multinodular growth pattern with prominent myxoid stromal change and numerous blood vessels
Giant cell fibroblastoma	• Pediatric variant of DFSP • Spindle cells with myxoid stroma, pseudovascular spaces lines with multinucleated giant cells
Sclerosing	• Rare variant • Sclerosis seen on histology
Atrophic	• Rare variant • Less cellular than classic DFSP
Fibrosarcomatous	• High-grade sarcomatous component that occupies 20%–80% of the tumor with the remaining areas with classic DFSP-type histology • Sarcomatous component cells are markedly atypical and more cellular • The presence of this variant increases tumor grade from low to intermediate • Impact on overall prognosis is unclear, but many studies show a higher rate of metastasis and worse prognosis

DFSP recurrence rate after MMS of 1.11% versus 6.32% after WLE.[39,48,55–57] For positive surgical margins or for DFSP recurrences, surgical resection is initially recommended; if not feasible, radiation therapy or imatinib chemotherapy should be considered.[51] DFSP is radiosensitive, but radiation is rarely the primary treatment unless the primary tumor is inoperable; it is used as adjuvant therapy after resection with positive margins.[58]

Imatinib, a tyrosine kinase inhibitor, is approved for treatment of DFSP with t(17;22). Imatinib is used for unresectable, recurrent, or metastatic DFSP.[30] Patients with locally advanced disease have responded fully to treatment with imatinib.[59] Limited data exist regarding other tyrosine kinase inhibitors and DFSP.[60,61] DFSP has a poor response to conventional chemotherapy.[62,63]

Prognosis and Follow-up

Overall prognosis for DFSP is excellent, with a 10-year survival of 99.1%.[32] Most recurrences occur within 3 years, but some develop after 5 years.[64,65] Given the possibility of recurrence or metastasis, follow-up is recommended every 6 to 12 months.[51]

Leiomyosarcoma

Superficial leiomyosarcomas (LMSs) are rare, indolent, malignant smooth muscle neoplasms subcategorized into primary dermal and primary subcutaneous forms. More aggressive LMS arises from even deeper soft tissues.[66] Dermal LMS rarely metastasizes, whereas subcutaneous LMS metastasizes in more than 25% of cases.[67,68]

Epidemiology

Cutaneous LMS comprises 4% to 6.5% of all soft tissue sarcomas, with an incidence of 0.2 per 100,000 per year.[69–72] Both subtypes occur in the fifth to eighth decade of life.[66,69,70,73] The dermal form overwhelmingly afflicts men, with equal gender occurrences of subcutaneous LMS.[69,70,74,75]

Pathogenesis

Dermal LMS is thought to originate from smooth muscle of the arrector pili, whereas subcutaneous LMS is thought to arise from vascular smooth muscle in subcutaneous adipose tissue. Each form can grow and extend to involve the subcutis or dermis.[69,70,73,76] Overexpression of receptor tyrosine kinases has been shown in some LMS.[77]

Clinical Features, Diagnosis, and Histology

Both dermal and subcutaneous LMS present like DFSP as subcutaneous skin-colored nodules or plaques; subcutaneous forms are typically larger. Both forms are usually asymptomatic (but can be painful) and usually occur on the extremities.[66,69,70,74,78,79] Although debate exists about whether dermal forms truly metastasize, subcutaneous forms have well-established metastatic potential (51%–62%).[66,69,72,74,80] Metastases involve cutaneous sites, lungs, liver, or brain.[66,76]

Tissue biopsy, either excisional or incisional, is required for diagnosis. Tumor depth provides important prognostic information; increasing depth correlates with worse outcomes.[75] On histology, LMS cells resemble smooth muscle cells but are atypical, with increased mitoses versus benign leiomyomas. Immunochemical stains of actin and desmin can aid in histologic diagnosis.[81]

Treatment

Obtaining clear histologic margins in LMS is paramount in preventing recurrence or metastasis. LMS can be excised with WLE or MMS or with MMS.[69,72,82–84] MMS is noted to have 0% recurrence and metastasis rates for superficial LMS, compared with 9% and 10% respectively for WLE.[66]

For unresectable or metastatic cases, chemotherapeutic regimens used in soft tissue sarcomas may be used. Limited data exist regarding targeted therapies with tyrosine kinase inhibitors.[71] In addition, the response to radiation therapy has been poor.[82,84–86]

Prognosis and Follow-up

Patients with superficial LMS require close follow-up. Average time to LMS metastasis is 5.6 years, with disease-specific mortality of dermal LMS of 6% and 40% for subcutaneous LMS.[76] Close follow-up for at least 5 to 10 years after diagnosis is recommended.[66]

SUMMARY

Cutaneous sarcomas, although rare, are important neoplastic diseases to recognize. Their heterogeneous physical findings and histologic appearance underscore the importance of clinicopathologic correlation in reaching accurate diagnoses. Efforts to characterize the molecular underpinnings giving rise to these neoplasms, as well as the most effective treatments for these rare malignancies, are currently the subject of ongoing translational investigations and clinical trials.

REFERENCES

1. Cohen JM, Burgin S. Moritz Kaposi: a notable name in dermatology. JAMA Dermatol 2015;151(8):867.

2. Hiatt KM, Nelson AM, Lichy JH, et al. Classic Kaposi sarcoma in the United States over the last two decades: a clinicopathologic and molecular study of 438 non-HIV-related Kaposi sarcoma patients with comparison to HIV-related Kaposi sarcoma. Mod Pathol 2008;21(5):572–82.

3. ARMSTRONG AW, LAM KH, CHASE EP. Epidemiology of classic and AIDS-related Kaposi's sarcoma in the USA: incidence, survival, and geographical distribution from 1975 to 2005. Epidemiol Infect 2013;141(01):200–6.

4. Royse KE, El Chaer F, Amirian ES, et al. Disparities in Kaposi sarcoma incidence and survival in the United States: 2000-2013. PLoS One 2017;12(8):e0182750.

5. Rabkin CS, Schulz TF, Whitby D, et al. Interassay correlation of human herpesvirus 8 serologic tests. HHV-8 Interlaboratory Collaborative Group. J Infect Dis 1998;178(2):304–9. Available at: http://www.ncbi.nlm.nih.gov/pubmed/9697708. Accessed July 8, 2018.

6. Gramolelli S, Schulz TF. The role of Kaposi sarcoma-associated herpesvirus in the pathogenesis of Kaposi sarcoma. J Pathol 2015;235(2):368–80.

7. Shiels MS, Islam JY, Rosenberg PS, et al. Projected cancer incidence rates and burden of incident cancer cases in HIV-infected adults in the United States through 2030. Ann Intern Med 2018;168(12):866.

8. Letang E, Lewis JJ, Bower M, et al. Immune reconstitution inflammatory syndrome associated with Kaposi sarcoma. AIDS 2013;27(10):1603–13.

9. Olweny CL, Kaddumukasa A, Atine I, et al. Childhood Kaposi's sarcoma: clinical features and therapy. Br J Cancer 1976;33(5):555–60. Available at: http://www.ncbi.nlm.nih.gov/pubmed/1276034. Accessed July 9, 2018.

10. Engels EA, Pfeiffer RM, Fraumeni JF, et al. Spectrum of cancer risk among US solid organ transplant recipients. JAMA 2011;306(17):1891–901.

11. Moosa MR. Racial and ethnic variations in incidence and pattern of malignancies after kidney transplantation. Medicine (Baltimore) 2005;84(1):12–22. Available at: http://www.ncbi.nlm.nih.gov/pubmed/15643296. Accessed July 9, 2018.

12. Euvrard S, Kanitakis J, Claudy A. Skin cancers after organ transplantation. N Engl J Med 2003;348(17):1681–91.

13. Grayson W, Pantanowitz L. Histological variants of cutaneous Kaposi sarcoma. Diagn Pathol 2008;3:31.

14. Singh NB, Lakier RH, Donde B. Hypofractionated radiation therapy in the treatment of epidemic Kaposi sarcoma – a prospective randomized trial. Radiother Oncol 2008;88(2):211–6.

15. Hauerstock D, Gerstein W, Vuong T. Results of radiation therapy for treatment of classic Kaposi sarcoma. J Cutan Med Surg 2009;13(1):18–21.

16. National Comprehensive Cancer Network. AIDS-related Kaposi sarcoma (Version 1.2018). 2017. Available at: https://www.nccn.org/professionals/physician_gls/pdf/kaposi.pdf. Accessed July 1, 2018.

17. Albores-Saavedra J, Schwartz AM, Henson DE, et al. Cutaneous angiosarcoma. Analysis of 434 cases from the surveillance, epidemiology, and end results program, 1973-2007. Ann Diagn Pathol 2011;15(2):93–7.

18. Leake J, Sheehan MP, Rampling D, et al. Angiosarcoma complicating xeroderma pigmentosum. Histopathology 1992;21(2):179–81. Available at: http://www.ncbi.nlm.nih.gov/pubmed/1505938. Accessed July 9, 2018.

19. Tomasini C, Grassi M, Pippione M. Cutaneous angiosarcoma arising in an irradiated breast. Case report and review of the literature. Dermatology 2004;209(3):208–14.

20. Anzalone CL, Cohen PR, Diwan AH, et al. Radiation-induced angiosarcoma. Dermatol Online J 2013;19(1):2. Available at: http://www.ncbi.nlm.nih.gov/pubmed/23374944. Accessed July 9, 2018.
21. Behjati S, Tarpey PS, Sheldon H, et al. Recurrent PTPRB and PLCG1 mutations in angiosarcoma. Nat Genet 2014;46(4):376–9.
22. Manner J, Radlwimmer B, Hohenberger P, et al. MYC high level gene amplification is a distinctive feature of angiosarcomas after irradiation or chronic lymphedema. Am J Pathol 2010;176(1):34–9.
23. Shustef E, Kazlouskaya V, Prieto VG, et al. Cutaneous angiosarcoma: a current update. J Clin Pathol 2017;70(11):917–25.
24. Suchak R, Thway K, Zelger B, et al. Primary cutaneous epithelioid angiosarcoma. Am J Surg Pathol 2011;35(1):60–9.
25. Guadagnolo BA, Zagars GK, Araujo D, et al. Outcomes after definitive treatment for cutaneous angiosarcoma of the face and scalp. Head Neck 2011;33(5):661–7.
26. Fujisawa Y, Yoshino K, Kadono T, et al. Chemoradiotherapy with taxane is superior to conventional surgery and radiotherapy in the management of cutaneous angiosarcoma: a multicentre, retrospective study. Br J Dermatol 2014;171(6):1493–500.
27. Ishida Y, Otsuka A, Kabashima K. Cutaneous angiosarcoma. Curr Opin Oncol 2017;30(2):1.
28. Sindhu S, Gimber LH, Cranmer L, et al. Angiosarcoma treated successfully with anti-PD-1 therapy - a case report. J Immunother Cancer 2017;5(1):58.
29. Gloster HM Jr. Dermatofibrosarcoma protuberans. J Am Acad Dermatol 1996;35(3 Pt 1):355–6.
30. Odueyungbo M, Ratner D. Update on the use and treatment of targeted molecular inhibitors for locally advanced and metastatic non-melanoma skin cancers. Dermatol Surg 2016;42(Suppl 1):S49–56.
31. Rouhani P, Fletcher CD, Devesa SS, et al. Cutaneous soft tissue sarcoma incidence patterns in the U.S.: an analysis of 12,114 cases. Cancer 2008;113(3):616–27.
32. Kreicher KL, Kurlander DE, Gittleman HR, et al. Incidence and survival of primary dermatofibrosarcoma protuberans in the United States. Dermatol Surg 2016;42(Suppl 1):S24–31.
33. Bowne WB, Antonescu CR, Leung DH, et al. Dermatofibrosarcoma protuberans: a clinicopathologic analysis of patients treated and followed at a single institution. Cancer 2000;88(12):2711–20.
34. Fiore M, Miceli R, Mussi C, et al. Dermatofibrosarcoma protuberans treated at a single institution: a surgical disease with a high cure rate. J Clin Oncol 2005;23(30):7669–75.
35. Sirvent N, Maire G, Pedeutour F. Genetics of dermatofibrosarcoma protuberans family of tumors: from ring chromosomes to tyrosine kinase inhibitor treatment. Genes Chromosomes Cancer 2003;37(1):1–19.
36. Navarro M, Simon MP, Migeon C, et al. COL1A1-PDGFB fusion in a ring chromosome 4 found in a dermatofibrosarcoma protuberans. Genes Chromosomes Cancer 1998;23(3):263–6.
37. Simon MP, Pedeutour F, Sirvent N, et al. Deregulation of the platelet-derived growth factor B-chain gene via fusion with collagen gene COL1A1 in dermatofibrosarcoma protuberans and giant-cell fibroblastoma. Nat Genet 1997;15(1):95–8.

38. Taylor HB, Helwig EB. Dermatofibrosarcoma protuberans. A study of 115 cases. Cancer 1962;15:717–25.
39. Bogucki B, Neuhaus I, Hurst EA. Dermatofibrosarcoma protuberans: a review of the literature. Dermatol Surg 2012;38(4):537–51.
40. Llombart B, Serra-Guillen C, Monteagudo C, et al. Dermatofibrosarcoma protuberans: a comprehensive review and update on diagnosis and management. Semin Diagn Pathol 2013;30(1):13–28.
41. Silverman JS, Tamsen A. CD34 and factor XIIIa-positive microvascular dendritic cells and the family of fibrohistiocytic mesenchymal tumors. Am J Dermatopathol 1998;20(5):533–6.
42. Abbott JJ, Oliveira AM, Nascimento AG. The prognostic significance of fibrosarcomatous transformation in dermatofibrosarcoma protuberans. Am J Surg Pathol 2006;30(4):436–43.
43. Ding J, Hashimoto H, Enjoji M. Dermatofibrosarcoma protuberans with fibrosarcomatous areas. A clinicopathologic study of nine cases and a comparison with allied tumors. Cancer 1989;64(3):721–9.
44. Mentzel T, Beham A, Katenkamp D, et al. Fibrosarcomatous ("high-grade") dermatofibrosarcoma protuberans: clinicopathologic and immunohistochemical study of a series of 41 cases with emphasis on prognostic significance. Am J Surg Pathol 1998;22(5):576–87.
45. Abdaljaleel MY, North JP. Sclerosing dermatofibrosarcoma protuberans shows significant overlap with sclerotic fibroma in both routine and immunohistochemical analysis: a potential diagnostic pitfall. Am J Dermatopathol 2017;39(2):83–8.
46. Criscione VD, Weinstock MA. Descriptive epidemiology of dermatofibrosarcoma protuberans in the United States, 1973 to 2002. J Am Acad Dermatol 2007;56(6): 968–73.
47. Liang CA, Jambusaria-Pahlajani A, Karia PS, et al. A systematic review of outcome data for dermatofibrosarcoma protuberans with and without fibrosarcomatous change. J Am Acad Dermatol 2014;71(4):781–6.
48. Foroozan M, Sei JF, Amini M, et al. Efficacy of Mohs micrographic surgery for the treatment of dermatofibrosarcoma protuberans: systematic review. Arch Dermatol 2012;148(9):1055–63.
49. Rutgers EJ, Kroon BB, Albus-Lutter CE, et al. Dermatofibrosarcoma protuberans: treatment and prognosis. Eur J Surg Oncol 1992;18(3):241–8.
50. Smola MG, Soyer HP, Scharnagl E. Surgical treatment of dermatofibrosarcoma protuberans. A retrospective study of 20 cases with review of literature. Eur J Surg Oncol 1991;17(5):447–53.
51. [on-line] NCCN (NCCN) G. Dermatofibrosarcoma protuberans (Version 1.2018). 2018. Available at: https://www.nccn.org/professionals/physician_gls/PDF/dfsp. pdf. Accessed July 1, 2018.
52. Acosta AE, Velez CS. Dermatofibrosarcoma protuberans. Curr Treat Options Oncol 2017;18(9):56.
53. Monnier D, Vidal C, Martin L, et al. Dermatofibrosarcoma protuberans: a population-based cancer registry descriptive study of 66 consecutive cases diagnosed between 1982 and 2002. J Eur Acad Dermatol Venereol 2006; 20(10):1237–42.
54. Reha J, Katz SC. Dermatofibrosarcoma protuberans. Surg Clin North Am 2016; 96(5):1031–46.
55. Paradisi A, Abeni D, Rusciani A, et al. Dermatofibrosarcoma protuberans: wide local excision vs. Mohs micrographic surgery. Cancer Treat Rev 2008;34(8): 728–36.

56. Thomas CJ, Wood GC, Marks VJ. Mohs micrographic surgery in the treatment of rare aggressive cutaneous tumors: the Geisinger experience. Dermatol Surg 2007;33(3):333–9.
57. Meguerditchian AN, Wang J, Lema B, et al. Wide excision or Mohs micrographic surgery for the treatment of primary dermatofibrosarcoma protuberans. Am J Clin Oncol 2010;33(3):300–3.
58. Williams N, Morris CG, Kirwan JM, et al. Radiotherapy for dermatofibrosarcoma protuberans. Am J Clin Oncol 2014;37(5):430–2.
59. McArthur GA, Demetri GD, van Oosterom A, et al. Molecular and clinical analysis of locally advanced dermatofibrosarcoma protuberans treated with imatinib: Imatinib Target Exploration Consortium Study B2225. J Clin Oncol 2005;23(4):866–73.
60. Kamar FG, Kairouz VF, Sabri AN. Dermatofibrosarcoma protuberans (DFSP) successfully treated with sorafenib: case report. Clin Sarcoma Res 2013;3(1):5.
61. Ong HS, Ji T, Wang LZ, et al. Dermatofibrosarcoma protuberans on the right neck with superior vena cava syndrome: case report and literature review. Int J Oral Maxillofac Surg 2013;42(6):707–10.
62. Labropoulos SV, Fletcher JA, Oliveira AM, et al. Sustained complete remission of metastatic dermatofibrosarcoma protuberans with imatinib mesylate. Anticancer Drugs 2005;16(4):461–6.
63. Ng A, Nishikawa H, Lander A, et al. Chemosensitivity in pediatric dermatofibrosarcoma protuberans. J Pediatr Hematol Oncol 2005;27(2):100–2.
64. Snow SN, Gordon EM, Larson PO, et al. Dermatofibrosarcoma protuberans: a report on 29 patients treated by Mohs micrographic surgery with long-term follow-up and review of the literature. Cancer 2004;101(1):28–38.
65. Chang CK, Jacobs IA, Salti GI. Outcomes of surgery for dermatofibrosarcoma protuberans. Eur J Surg Oncol 2004;30(3):341–5.
66. Winchester DS, Hocker TL, Brewer JD, et al. Leiomyosarcoma of the skin: clinical, histopathologic, and prognostic factors that influence outcomes. J Am Acad Dermatol 2014;71(5):919–25.
67. Svarvar C, Bohling T, Berlin O, et al. Clinical course of nonvisceral soft tissue leiomyosarcoma in 225 patients from the Scandinavian Sarcoma Group. Cancer 2007;109(2):282–91.
68. Hornick JL, Fletcher CD. Criteria for malignancy in nonvisceral smooth muscle tumors. Ann Diagn Pathol 2003;7(1):60–6.
69. Bernstein SC, Roenigk RK. Leiomyosarcoma of the skin. Treatment of 34 cases. Dermatol Surg 1996;22(7):631–5.
70. Fields JP, Helwig EB. Leiomyosarcoma of the skin and subcutaneous tissue. Cancer 1981;47(1):156–69.
71. Kohlmeyer J, Steimle-Grauer SA, Hein R. Cutaneous sarcomas. J Dtsch Dermatol Ges 2017;15(6):630–48.
72. Fauth CT, Bruecks AK, Temple W, et al. Superficial leiomyosarcoma: a clinicopathologic review and update. J Cutan Pathol 2010;37(2):269–76.
73. Phelan JT, Sherer W, Mesa P. Malignant smooth-muscle tumors (leiomyosarcomas) of soft-tissue origin. N Engl J Med 1962;266:1027–30.
74. Dahl I, Angervall L. Cutaneous and subcutaneous leiomyosarcoma. A clinicopathologic study of 47 patients. Pathol Eur 1974;9(4):307–15.
75. Jensen ML, Jensen OM, Michalski W, et al. Intradermal and subcutaneous leiomyosarcoma: a clinicopathological and immunohistochemical study of 41 cases. J Cutan Pathol 1996;23(5):458–63.

76. Winchester DS, Hocker TL, Roenigk RK. Skin metastases of leiomyosarcoma (LMS): a retrospective review of 21 cases. J Am Acad Dermatol 2015;72(5): 910–2.
77. Luke JJ, Keohan ML. Advances in the systemic treatment of cutaneous sarcomas. Semin Oncol 2012;39(2):173–83.
78. Massi D, Franchi A, Alos L, et al. Primary cutaneous leiomyosarcoma: clinicopathological analysis of 36 cases. Histopathology 2010;56(2):251–62.
79. Kaddu S, Beham A, Cerroni L, et al. Cutaneous leiomyosarcoma. Am J Surg Pathol 1997;21(9):979–87.
80. Kraft S, Fletcher CD. Atypical intradermal smooth muscle neoplasms: clinicopathologic analysis of 84 cases and a reappraisal of cutaneous "leiomyosarcoma". Am J Surg Pathol 2011;35(4):599–607.
81. Holst VA, Junkins-Hopkins JM, Elenitsas R. Cutaneous smooth muscle neoplasms: clinical features, histologic findings, and treatment options. J Am Acad Dermatol 2002;46(4):477–90 [quiz: 491–4].
82. Starling J 3rd, Coldiron BM. Mohs micrographic surgery for the treatment of cutaneous leiomyosarcoma. J Am Acad Dermatol 2011;64(6):1119–22.
83. Humphreys TR, Finkelstein DH, Lee JB. Superficial leiomyosarcoma treated with Mohs micrographic surgery. Dermatol Surg 2004;30(1):108–12.
84. Deneve JL, Messina JL, Bui MM, et al. Cutaneous leiomyosarcoma: treatment and outcomes with a standardized margin of resection. Cancer Control 2013; 20(4):307–12.
85. Tsutsumida A, Yoshida T, Yamamoto Y, et al. Management of superficial leiomyosarcoma: a retrospective study of 10 cases. Plast Reconstr Surg 2005;116(1): 8–12.
86. Porter CJ, Januszkiewicz JS. Cutaneous leiomyosarcoma. Plast Reconstr Surg 2002;109(3):964–7.

Mycosis Fungoides and Sézary Syndrome: An Update

Cecilia Larocca, MD*, Thomas Kupper, MD

KEYWORDS

- Mycosis fungoides • Sézary syndrome • Cutaneous T-cell lymphoma • Review
- Diagnosis • Genetics • Therapy • Cause

KEY POINTS

- Mycosis fungoides and Sézary syndrome are the most common non-Hodgkin lymphomas to arise from skin-tropic clonal T lymphocytes.
- Significant advances have been made in understanding the genetic and epigenetic aberrations in mycosis fungoides and Sézary syndrome.
- Diagnosis requires a combination of clinical, pathologic, and molecular features.
- Several prognostic factors have been recognized to identify patients with poor prognosis.
- Treatment is intended to minimize morbidity and limit disease progression, as cure is rarely achieved.

INTRODUCTION

Cutaneous T-cell lymphomas (CTCLs) encompass a heterogeneous collection of non-Hodgkin lymphomas that arise from skin-tropic memory T lymphocytes. Among them, mycosis fungoides (MF) and Sézary syndrome (SS) are the most common malignancies. In its earliest stages, patients classically present with discrete skin lesions that resemble eczema or with widespread erythema. Patients with advanced disease may have fungating tumors or leukemic disease with eventual involvement of lymph nodes and viscera. Most patients with MF present with early stage disease and have an indolent disease course with a low risk of disease progression; however, cure is rarely achieved. The goal of treatment is to minimize symptomatic morbidity and limit disease progression. Increasingly, hematopoietic stem cell transplantation is being considered for patients with advanced stages, is the only therapy with curative intent.

EPIDEMIOLOGY

The overall incidence of CTCL is 10.2 per million persons.[1] More than half of these cases are MF, with an incidence of 5.6 per million persons.[1] The age-adjusted

Department of Dermatology, Brigham and Women's Hospital, Dana Farber Cancer Institute, Harvard Medical School, 450 Brookline Avenue, Boston, MA 02115, USA
* Corresponding author.
E-mail address: clarocca@bwh.harvard.edu

Hematol Oncol Clin N Am 33 (2019) 103–120
https://doi.org/10.1016/j.hoc.2018.09.001
0889-8588/19/© 2018 Elsevier Inc. All rights reserved.

incidence rate for SS is 0.1 per million persons.[2] Men are more commonly affected than women (incidence rate ratio [IRR] = 1.6).[2] The incidence increases with age, with the highest CTCL incidence at greater than 70 years of age. Blacks have a higher incidence rate than whites (IRR = 1.57).[2] Black patients are diagnosed at an earlier age (median age of diagnosis of 53 years, compared with 63 years for whites) and have worse survival than white patients regardless of age and stage of presentation.[2]

DIAGNOSIS

The diagnosis of MF/SS can be challenging and requires input from the clinical presentation, pathologic evaluation, and molecular studies. MF/SS can resemble benign inflammatory dermatoses, and characteristic histologic features of MF may be absent in early disease even after multiple biopsies. Moreover, traditional polymerase chain reaction (PCR) of the T-cell receptor (TCR) used to identify the presence of a T-cell clone in clinical samples has a significant false-negative rate in early stage disease.[3] An algorithm to assist in the diagnosis of early MF has been proposed, although not formally validated.[4] This algorithm emphasizes the importance of integrating the clinical presentation (persistent, progressive patches or plaques in non–sun-exposed location and morphology), histopathology (superficial lymphoid infiltrate, epidermotropism without spongiosis, lymphoid atypia), immunopathology (decreased expression of CD5, CD7 or epidermal-dermal discordance of CD2, CD3, CD5, CD7), and molecular evaluation of T-cell clonality.[4] Pathologic criteria to assist in the diagnosis have been put forth but are not often used in clinical practice.[5] To date there are no diagnostic molecular markers used clinically that can reliably identify malignant T-cell from benign T-cell. However, expression of TOX, a thymocyte selection-associated HMG box protein, may be a useful adjunct.[6–8]

There are 3 clinical morphologies in MF: patch, plaque, and tumor (**Fig. 1–3**).[9,10] Each is distinguished from the former by increasing thickness. There are 3 recognized

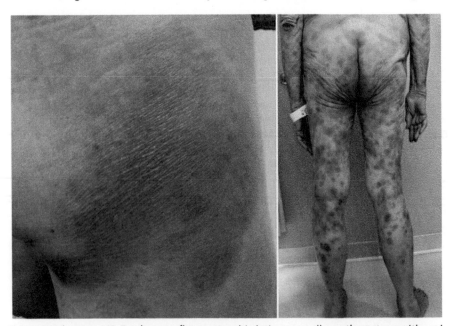

Fig. 1. Patch-stage MF. Patches are flat to atrophic lesions, usually erythematous with variable amounts of scale, and may resemble eczema. Atrophic lesions have a cigarette-paper, wrinkled appearance. (*Courtesy of* J. O'Malley, MD, PhD, Boston, MA.)

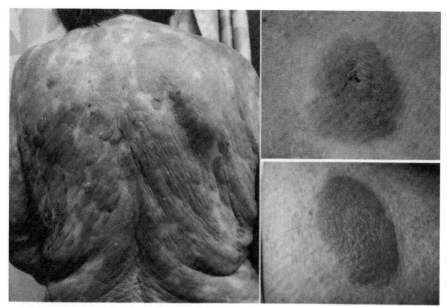

Fig. 2. Plaque-stage MF. Plaques are raised or indurated lesions. Affected acral sites are considered plaques.

subtypes of MF by the World Health Organization(WHO)/European Organization for Research and Treatment of Cancer (EORTC) with different clinical and histologic features (**Table 1, Fig. 4**).[11] Clinicians must also be aware of the several distinct clinicopathologic variants of MF (**Box 1, Fig. 5**).[12]

Patients with SS typically present with erythroderma, defined as diffuse erythema affecting at least 80% of the body surface area (**Fig. 6**).[11] These patients must be distinguished from other benign causes of erythroderma (**Box 2**).

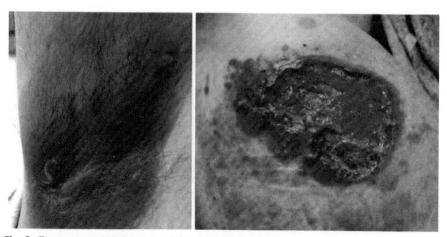

Fig. 3. Tumor-stage MF. Tumors exhibit a significant vertical growth phase and must measure at least 1 cm in diameter. They are often ulcerated.

Table 1
Mycosis fungoides variants recognized by the World Health Organization/European Organization for Research and Treatment of Cancer

MF Subtype	Clinical Presentation	Immunophenotype	Histology
Folliculotropic MF	Predilection for head/neck Alopecic skin lesions Follicular papules; Acneiform/comedonal-like papules or nodules (see **Fig. 4**)	CD4+CD3+ T-cell Admixed CD30 + blasts	Perivascular and periadenexal lymphocytic infiltrates with infiltration of follicular epithelium (folliculotropism); variable infiltration of eccrine sweat glands by atypical lymphocytes with sparing of epidermis; follicular mucinosis
Pagetoid reticulosis	Predilection for extremities Localized psoriasiform patch or plaque Indolent clinical behavior	CD4+CD3+ T-cell or CD8+CD3+ T-cell CD30 often positive	Hyperplastic epithelium with marked pagetoid-like atypical lymphocytes; dermis with mixed reactive lymphocytes and histiocytes
Granulomatous slack skin	Predilection from axillae and groin Lax pendulous skin Indolent clinical behavior	CD4+CD3+ T-cell	Dense granulomatous dermal infiltrates of atypical lymphocytes, macrophages, many multinucleated giants cells; destruction of elastic tissue

Data from Willemze R, Jaffe ES, Burg G, et al. WHO-EORTC classification for cutaneous lymphomas. Blood 2005;105(10):3768–85.

The single greatest advancement to aid in the diagnosis of MF/SS is the advent of high-throughput sequencing (HTS) of the TCRB gene, which permits identification of a T-cell clone through the sequence of its CDR3 region with superior sensitivity compared with traditional *TCRG* PCR (**Fig. 7**).[3] It has also shown to be effective at discriminating between CTCL and benign inflammatory diseases when the frequency of the top T-cell clone is evaluated as the fraction of total nucleated cells.[3] This analysis, however, is being used in a limited number of cancer centers at this time.

Given these diagnostic challenges, referral of patients to specialized multidisciplinary cutaneous lymphoma cancer centers is advised.

STAGING AND PROGNOSIS

Staging of MF/SS was initially set forth by the MF Cooperative Group of the American Joint Committee on Cancer.[9] The International Society for Cutaneous Lymphomas

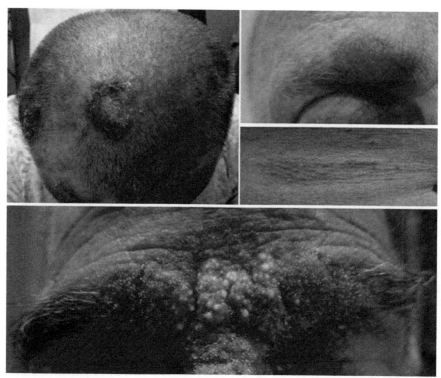

Fig. 4. Folliculotropic MF. Lesions preferentially affect the head and neck area. When located within hair-bearing areas, it may cause alopecia. Patches or plaques may be composed of cyst-like or follicular-based papules.

(ISCL) and the EORTC in 2007 proposed a revision of the staging criteria, which was later validated in a single-center cohort of 1502 patients.[9] The National Comprehensive Cancer Network (NCCN) has adapted the revised ISCL/EORTC recommendations for staging of MF/SS (**Tables 2–4**).

Box 1
Clinicopathologic variants of mycosis fungoides

MF clinical variants
  Bullous
  Hypopigmented (see **Fig. 5**)
  Ichthyosiform
  MF palmaris et plantaris (keratoderma-like)
  Pigmented purpuric dermatosis-like
  Papular
  Poikilodermatous
  Psoriasiform
  Pustular
  Solitary/unilesional
  Syringotropic
  Verrucoid

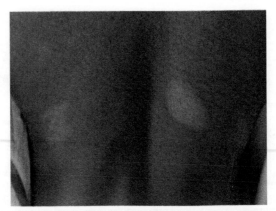

Fig. 5. Hypopigmented MF. Predominately affects African Americans. It has an indolent disease course. Immunophenotype is classically of atypical CD8+ T-cell.

Clinical stage is an important determinant of the risk of disease progression (RDP) and overall survival (OS).[13] Patients with stage IA have a median survival of 35.5 years and a disease-specific survival (DSS) of 90% at 20 years, which is comparable with patients without MF. Although these patients have an indolent disease course, there is an 18% RDP at 20 years.[13] Patients with stage IB have a median survival of 21.5 years, a DSS of 67%, and an RDP of 47% at 20 years.[13] Patients with stage IIA have a median survival of 15.8 years, a DSS of 60%, and an RDP 41% at 20 years.[13] Patients with stage IIB have a median survival of 4.7 years and a DSS of 56% at 5 years and 29% at 20 years.[13] Their RDP is 48% by 5 years and 71% by 20 years.[13] Patients with IIIA and IIIB have a median survival of 4.7 and 3.4 years, respectively, and a 10-year DSS of 45%.[13] Their RDP is 53% and 82%, respectively.[13] Patients with stage IVA1 have a median survival of 3.8 years, a DSS of 41% at 5 years and 20% at 10 years.[13] Their RDP is 62% at 5 years.[13] Patients with stage IVA2 have a median survival of 2.1 years and a DSS of 23% at 5 years and 20% at 10 years.[13] Their RDP is 77% by 5 years.[13] Patients with stage IVB have a median survival of 1.4 years with a DSS of 18% at 5 years.[13]

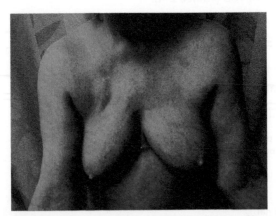

Fig. 6. Erythroderma. Erythroderma is defined as diffuse erythema affecting 80% or greater body surface areas. It often appears eczematous with a variable amount of scale. Erythroderma is often a sign of leukemic disease.

> **Box 2**
> **Causes of erythroderma**
>
> Differential diagnosis of erythroderma
>   Idiopathic
>   Atopic dermatitis
>   Psoriasis
>   Pityriasis rubra pilaris
>   SS
>   Systemic allergic contact dermatitis

In this patient cohort, several prognostic factors were identified.[13] Advanced age was associated with a higher RDP, poorer OS, and worse DSS. Skin (T) stage, B0b (compared with those with B0a), folliculotropic MF, large-cell transformation (LCT), and elevated lactate dehydrogenase (LDH) were independently associated with RDP, worse OS, and DSS. These prognostic factors gave rise to the prognostic index score, developed by the Cutaneous Lymphoma International Consortium study, for patients with advanced MF/SS.[14] Stage IV, age greater than 60 years, large-cell transformation, and increased LDH were combined into a 3-tier prognostic index model. These risk groups had significantly different 5-year survival rates regardless of patient stage (IIB–IV): low risk (68%), intermediate risk (44%), and high risk (28%).

One of the greatest challenges in the management of MF is the identification of which early stage patients are at risk for disease progression. A significant advancement in identify these patients comes from the work of de Masson and colleagues.[15] In this single-center retrospective study, the burden of malignant T-cell clone (tumor clone frequency [TCF]) in lesional skin predicted RDP and OS in early stage patients. A TCF of greater than 25% was significantly associated with progression-free survival (PFS) and OS. This measure was superior to predicting the PFS compared with stage (IB vs IA), presence of plaques, elevated LDH, age, and the presence of LCT. Furthermore, when patients at high risk of disease progression as determined by TCF were treated with radiation, a superior therapy capable of locally eliminating malignant disease, they had an improved OS (O'Malley and colleagues, submitted for publication).

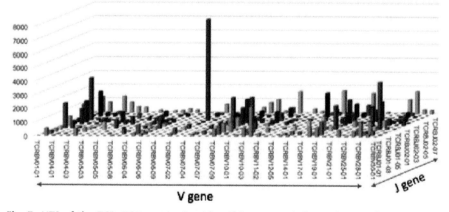

Fig. 7. HTS of the TCR. TCR sequencing identifying expanded population of clonal malignant T-cell in a patient with patch-stage CTCL. The V versus J gene usages of T-cell from a patch MF lesion are shown. The gray peak includes the clonal malignant T-cell population and other benign T-cell that share the same V and J usage. (Image *courtesy of* Dr. John O'Malley.)

Table 2
International Society for Cutaneous Lymphomas/European Organization for Research and Treatment of Cancer classification of mycosis fungoides/Sézary syndrome

TNMB Stages	Definition
T (Skin)	
T1	Patches, papules, and/or plaques covering <10% BSA T1a patch only T1b plaque ± patch
T2	Patches, papules, and/or plaques covering ≥10% BSA T2a patch only T2b plaque ± patch
T3	One or more tumors (at least one 1-cm-diameter solid or nodular lesion with evidence of depth and/or vertical growth
T4	Confluence of erythema covering ≥80% BSA
N (Node)	
N0	No clinically abnormal peripheral lymph nodes, biopsy not required
N1	Clinically abnormal peripheral lymph nodes, histopathology Dutch grade 1 or NCI LN_{0-2} N1a clone negative N1b clone positive
N2	Clinically abnormal peripheral lymph nodes, histopathology Dutch grade 2 or NCI LN_3 N2a clone negative N2b clone positive
N3	Clinically abnormal peripheral lymph nodes, histopathology Dutch grade 3–4 or NCI LN_4, clone positive or negative
Nx	Clinically abnormal peripheral lymph nodes, no histopathologic confirmation
Visceral (M)	
M0	No visceral organ involvement
M1	Visceral involvement (must have pathology, and organ is to be specified)
Blood	
B0	Absence of significant blood involvement: ≤5% of blood lymphocytes are Sézary cells B0a clone negative B0b clone positive
B1	Low blood tumor burden: >5% of peripheral blood lymphocytes are Sézary cells but does not meet criteria for B2 disease B1a clone negative B1b clone positive
B2*	High blood tumor burden: ≥100/uL Sézary cells with positive clone in blood (matching clone in skin) or positive clone and one of the following: 1. CD4/CD8 ratio of 10 or more 2. ≥40% CD4+CD7- cells of total lymphocytes 3. ≥30% CD4+CD26- cells of total lymphocytes

Abbreviation: BSA, body surface area.

Republished with permission of American Society of Hematology, from Olsen E, Vonderheid E, Pimpinelli N, et al. Revisions to the staging and classification of mycosis fungoides and Sezary syndrome: a proposal of the International Society for Cutaneous Lymphomas (ISCL) and the cutaneous lymphoma task force of the European Organization of Research and Treatment of Cancer (EORTC). Blood 2007;110(6):1715; permission conveyed through Copyright Clearance Center, Inc.

Table 3
Histopathologic staging of lymph nodes

Classification	Dutch System	NCI Classification
N1	Grade 1: Dermatopathic lymphadenopathy	LN0: No atypical lymphocytes LN1: Occasional, isolated atypical lymphocytes LN2: many atypical lymphocytes in 3–6 cell clusters
N2	Grade2: Dermatopathic lymphadenopathy, early involvement of MF	LN3: Aggregates of atypical lymphocytes; nodal architecture preserved
N3	Grade 3: Partial effacement of LN architecture; many atypical cells Grade 4: Complete effacement	LN4: Partial to complete effacement of nodal architecture by atypical lymphocytes

Determination of malignant clonal burden by HTS has also been found important in determining outcomes following bone marrow transplantation.[16]

PATHOPHYSIOLOGY
Malignant T-Cell Origin

Although MF and SS have overlapping presentations and are not distinguished in the WHO/EORTC staging criteria, they are considered separate entities.[11] The WHO/EORTC and the ISCL consider SS to be a clinical syndrome presenting with erythrodermic skin and leukemic disease.[9] This consideration is in contrast to patients who initially present with classic skin lesions of MF and later meet the staging criteria for

Table 4
World Health Organization/European Organization for Research and Treatment of Cancer staging of mycosis fungoides/Sézary syndrome

Stage	T	N	M	B
IA	1.0	0	0	0.1
IB	2.0	0	0	0.1
II	1.2	1.2	0	0.1
IIB	3.0	0–2	0	0.1
IIIA	4.0	0–2	0	0
IIIB	4.0	0–2	0	1.0
IVA1	1–4	0–2	0	2.0
IVA2	1–4	3.0	0	0–2
IVB	1–4	0–3	1	0–2

SS. The latter are referred to as leukemic MF, SS preceded by MF, or secondary SS. The NCCN considers patients with SS to be anyone who meets the criteria for a high blood burden of disease (B2 disease).

MF and SS classically arise from skin tropic memory CD4+ T-cell (CD8+ and CD4–CD8- subtypes may also be observed); but demonstration of different T-cell surface phenotypes and molecular profiles support the hypothesis that these malignancies originate from distinct memory T-cell subsets: the skin resident memory T-cell (T_{RM}) in MF and the skin-tropic central memory T-cell (T_{CM}) in SS.[17]

The average adult skin contains about 20 billion T-cell.[18] These T-cell are normally present in noninflamed human skin.[19] Most of these T-cell are memory T-cell; less than 5% are naïve.[18] Naïve T-cell reside in the blood or lymph nodes.[20] If naïve T-cell first encounter antigen in skin-draining lymph nodes, they proliferate clonally as effector T-cell and differentiate to express the skin homing addressin cutaneous lymphocyte antigen (CLA) and the C-C chemokine receptor 4 (CCR4) (**Fig. 8**).[20] Once these effector T-cell eliminate their cognate antigen, they differentiate into memory T-cell (**Fig. 8**).[20–22] Skin T_{CM} cells are CCR4+/CCR7+/L-selectin+, which allows for circulation in skin, blood, and lymph nodes.[22] Skin resident T_{RM} cells are CCR4+/CLA+ and lack CCR7 and L-selectin. They rarely circulate out of the skin.[22] A subset of T-cell, termed the migratory memory T-cell (T_{MM}), express CCR7 but not L-selectin and perhaps represent an intermediate phenotype recirculating more slowly out of the skin to blood compared with the T_{CM}.[22,23]

Campbell and colleagues[17] showed that MF malignant T-cell are CCR4+/CLA+/L-selectin-/CCR7- (T_{RM}), whereas SS malignant T-cell are CCR4+/L-selectin+/CCR7+ (T_{CM}). The molecular behavior of these T-cell types correlates with the clinical presentation of their malignant counterpart (**Fig. 9**). Skin T_{RM} are nonmigratory populations, and clinically patients with MF have fixed skin lesions with discrete borders.[20,24] In contrast, T_{CM} recirculate between skin, blood, and lymph node; clinically patients with SS have diffuse erythema and leukemic disease.[17,23] Patients with a T_{MM} phenotype have ill-defined but discrete skin lesions.[22,23] Interestingly, patients with a T_{MM} phenotype do not respond to alemtuzumab as well as patients with a T_{CM} phenotype. This therapy is effective only for leukemic disease; malignant T_{CM} cells seem to recirculate into frequently.[23]

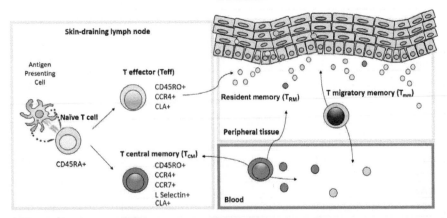

Fig. 8. Skin-tropic T-cell subtypes. Naïve T-cell differentiate into effector memory and central memory T-cell after binding to their cognate antigen on antigen presenting cells in skin-draining lymph nodes. Expression of surface ligand CCR4 determines their skin homing ability. Expression of CCR7/L-selectin determines their ability to re-circulate between blood and lymph node.

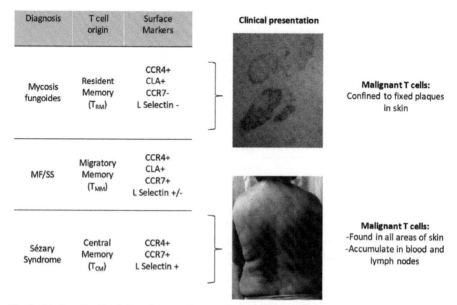

Diagnosis	T cell origin	Surface Markers	Clinical presentation
Mycosis fungoides	Resident Memory (T_{RM})	CCR4+ CLA+ CCR7- L Selectin -	**Malignant T cells:** Confined to fixed plaques in skin
MF/SS	Migratory Memory (T_{MM})	CCR4+ CLA+ CCR7+ L Selectin +/-	
Sézary Syndrome	Central Memory (T_{CM})	CCR4+ CCR7+ L Selectin +	**Malignant T cells:** -Found in all areas of skin -Accumulate in blood and lymph nodes

Fig. 9. Distinct T-cell origins of MF and SS. Surface molecular phenotype correlates with clinical presentation and morphology of skin disease. T_{MM}, migratory memory T-cell.

Genomic Alterations

MF/SS have diverse and complex genomic abnormalities, which have been best studied in SS. Striking findings include the discovery of many chromosomal abnormalities; somatic copy number variations (SCNVs) are favored over single nucleotide variants (SNVs) with 92% of all driver mutations arising from SCNVs.[25] Chromosomal aberrations most often occur on chromosomes 8, 10, and 17.[25–27] There is a high incidence of complex chromosomal structural rearrangements with more than 65% of patient samples exhibiting at least one chromothripsis-like rearrangement.[25] Chromosomal instability may be favored because of abnormal DNA repair machinery, activation of RAG endonucleases, impaired cell cycle control, and widespread DNA hypomethylation.[25,28,29] Most (74%) point mutations are C > T because of age-related and UVB-related mutagenesis.[25]

A meta-analysis of 220 genetically profiled patients with CTCL identified 55 driver mutations and implicated 14 biologically relevant pathways.[28] Affected pathways broadly include those involved in T-cell activation, function, migration, and differentiation; chromatin modification; cell cycle, survival and proliferation; and DNA damage response (**Table 5**).[25–28,30] Most genes are affected because of SCNV.[25,30] Mutations within genes are comparably much less common across CTCL cohorts (**Table 6**).[27,31]

It is not surprising given the recurrent alterations of epigenetic modifiers that patients with SS exhibit marked hypomethylation and hypermethylation of CpG islands across the genome compared with patients with benign inflammatory dermatoses and solid tumor malignancies.[29] Overall the SS methylome is most comparable with that of regulatory T-cell.[29] Evaluation of open chromatin sites used to predict transcription factor binding sites in CTCL samples, using assay of transposase-accessible chromatin with sequencing, showed unique regulomes and chromatin dynamics in CTCL cells compared with benign host T-cell and healthy donor T-cell.[32] Notable findings include decreased interferon gamma, interleukin (IL)-2, NFAT, and

Table 5
Pathways affected in mycosis fungoides/Sézary syndrome

Biological Pathway	Affected Gene/Pathway
T-cell function, cytokine signaling	CD28, CARD11, PDCD1, PLCG1, RLTPR, PTPRN2, PRKCB, PRKCQ, CSNK1A1, CCR4, ZEB4, JAK1/2/3, STAT3/5B, TNFRSF1B, NFKB2, IRF4
Chromatin modification	ARID1A, DNMT3A, KMT2C, KMT2D, SETDB2, TRRAP, TET1/2, KDM6A, NCOR1, BCOR, SMARCB1, CTCF
Cell cycle, survival, and proliferation	CDKN2A, CDKN1A, CDK4, MYC, RB1, RPSKA1, FAS, MAPK, and PI3K-Akt pathways
DNA damage response	TP53, ATM

PIK3R1 (regulatory subunit of PI3K) expression in leukemic cells and gain of expression of HDAC9 and natural killer–kB in all samples with activation of 1 of 3 transcription factor motif patterns due to chromatin modification: Jun-AP1; CTCF; or EGR, SMAD, MYC, and KLF.[32] Interestingly, differences in the chromatin accessibility landscape among leukemic cells predicted responses to HDAC inhibitors.[32]

Immunopathogenesis

Patients with MF/SS are at increased risk of bacterial infection, especially in advanced stages, because of the disruption of the skin barrier by ulcerated tumors as well as depressed local and systemic immune response to pathogens.[33] Immunosuppression is directly correlated with the malignant T-cell burden and is driven in part by abnormalities in the JAK/STAT signaling pathway (**Fig. 10**).[27,34,35] The tumor microenvironment becomes skewed from a T-helper 1 to a T-helper 2 phenotype with advancing stages.[34,36–38] These effects are reversible with depletion of malignant T-cell.[39]

Cause

Although the cause of MF is unknown, the leading therapy is the chronic antigen stimulation theory first described in 1974 by Tan and colleagues.[40] Chronic antigen or superantigen stimulation is thought to lead to clonal expansion of T-cell and malignant transformation. Several lines of observation support this theory. MF/SS is largely a malignancy of memory T-cell.[17] Malignant T-cell depend on dendritic cells for survival and proliferation.[41] The most frequent clonally expanded TCR vβ gene is TRBV20 to 1, which is associated with recognition of Staphylococcus aureus.[27] S aureus, in a series of patients with MF/SS, was able to act as a superantigen

Table 6	
Recurrently affected genes in mycosis fungoides/Sézary syndrome	
Affected by CNV (% of CTCL Samples)	**Affected by SNV (% of CTCL Samples)**
TP53 (92.5%)	MLL3 (4%–57%)
ZEB1 (65%)	TP53 (16%–43%)
STAT5B (63%)	ZEB1 (4%–27%)
ARID1A (58%)	STAT5B (2.77%–26.0%)
CDKN2A (40%)	ARID1A (8%–25%)
FAS (40%)	CARD11 (7%–22%)
DNMT3A (38%)	FAS (3%–19%)
ATM (30%)	PLCG1 (18%)
PRKCQ (30%)	CDKN2A (4%–17%)
TNFAIP3 (25%)	

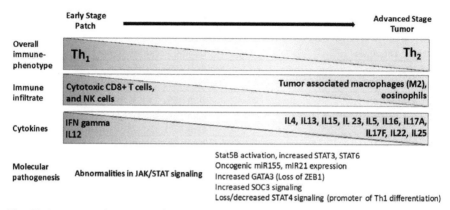

Fig. 10. Immunopathogenesis of MF/SS.

and stimulate proliferation of malignant T-cell.[42] As yet, no heritable germ-line mutations have been identified. However, patients with psoriasis and atopic dermatitis, which has a known familial inheritance, are at a somewhat higher risk for MF/SS.[43,44] Most patients with CTCL, however, have no antecedent T-cell–mediated skin disease. Many infectious agents have been investigated for putative roles in the cause of MF/SS. However, the data are limited and studies have yielded contradictory results to reliably implicate any single infectious agent, including HTLV-1 in CTCL.[45,46] Recently, a more sophisticated genomic analysis of SS samples using VirCapSeq-VERT revealed no functional coding sequences for viral pathogens or unknown viruses or evidence for active infection.[47] Interestingly, partially coding proviral sequences of human endogenous retroviruses (HERVs) were detected.[47] Although these particles may play a pathogenic role in disease, given that HERVs are normally present in the human genome, demonstrating a causal role in CTCL will be challenging.[48]

TREATMENT

Treatment is often multidisciplinary, as it combines skin-directed (**Table 7**) and systemic therapies (**Table 8**). Although there are several therapies recognized

Table 7
Skin-directed therapies for the treatment of mycosis fungoides/Sézary syndrome

Skin-Directed Therapies	Overall Response Rate (%)
Topical superpotent corticosteroids	75–95
Bexarotene gel	50–75
Nitrogen mustard/mechlorethamine HCl gel	50–90
Imiquimod cream	50
Tazarotene cream	58
Narrow-band UVB	54–90
PUVA	85–100
Radiation therapy (local external electron beam, brachytherapy, total skin electron beam therapy)	—

Abbreviations: HCl, hydrochloride; PUVA, psoralen UVA.

Table 8
Systemic therapies used to treat mycosis fungoides/Sézary syndrome

Systemic Therapies	Overall Response Rate
Bexarotene	ORR 45%, CR 13%[14]
IFN α	ORR 64%; CR 27% in stage IA–IVA[15]
Romidepsin	ORR 38%, CR 6%[16]
Methotrexate	ORR 58%, CR 41% in erythrodermic MF[17] ORR 33%, CR 12% in plaque-stage MF[18]
Brentuximab vedotin	ORR 65%, CR 10%[10]
Pralatrexate	ORR 41%, CR <1%[19]
Doxorubicin	ORR 30% to 80%, CR 20% to 60%[20,21]
Gemcitabine	ORR 51.0%–70.5%, CR 11.5%–23.0%[22,23]
Pembrolizumab	ORR 38%, 1 CR[24]
Bortezomib	ORR 67%, CR 17%[25]

Abbreviations: IFN, interferon; ORR, overall response rate.

by the NCCN for the treatment of MF/SS, there is a paucity of effective therapies providing durable responses. Targeted therapies have variable response rates ranging from 30% to 67%, with complete responses no higher than 41%.[49–61]

Furthermore, although traditional chemotherapy may have a higher response rate, these gains are short-lived and associated with worse overall outcomes.[62–64] Traditional nonmyeloablative allogeneic stem cell transplantation, the only potential cure for CTCL, has a 46% OS at 5 years.[65] Recently, the Stanford transplantation regimen showed an overall response rate of 90% with a 2-year OS and PFS of 76% and 50%, respectively.[66] There was a low incidence of graft-versus-host disease (GVHD) (23% grade II–IV acute GVHD and 23% with chronic GVHD at 2 years). Nonrelapse mortality due to GVHD or secondary malignancy at 1 year was 3%.[66] An important predictor of successful transplantation is the degree of remission achieved before transplant. Because CR is more readily achieve in SS than in advanced MF, most successful transplants have been performed in patients with SS.

Given the limited efficacy of existing therapies, patients with advanced disease are encouraged to participate in clinical trials. Several agents are in clinical development for the treatment of MF/SS (**Table 9**).

Table 9
Therapies in clinical development for cutaneous T-cell lymphoma

Investigational Agent	Clinical Development
Mogamulizumab (anti-CCR4 antibody)	Phase III (NCT01728805)
E7777 (cytotoxic IL-2 fusion protein)	Phase II (NCT01871727)
MRG-106 (miR-155 antagonist)	Phase II (NCT02580552)
Duvelisib (PI3K inhibitor)	Phase II (NCT02783625)
Ruxolitinib (JAK 1/2 inhibitor)	Phase II (NCT02974647)
TTI-621 (SIRPaFc IgG4, anti-CD47)	Phase I (NCT02663518)

SUMMARY

This is an exciting time in cutaneous oncology. The advent of HTS for TCR has enhanced our ability to diagnose MF/SS earlier, to predict which patients are at risk for disease progression, and to predict the treatment response to bone marrow transplantation. Major insights into disease biology have been made through genomic and epigenomic studies of MF/SS. There are increasing numbers of clinical trials for novel therapies for MF/SS.

REFERENCES

1. Korgavkar K, Xiong M, Weinstock M. Changing incidence trends of cutaneous T-cell lymphoma. JAMA Dermatol 2013;149(11):1295–9.
2. Imam MH, Shenoy PJ, Flowers CR, et al. Incidence and survival patterns of cutaneous T-cell lymphomas in the United States. Leuk Lymphoma 2013;54(4):752–9.
3. Kirsch IR, Watanabe R, O'Malley JT, et al. TCR sequencing facilitates diagnosis and identifies mature T cells as the cell of origin in CTCL. Sci Transl Med 2015; 7(308):308ra158.
4. Pimpinelli N, Olsen EA, Santucci M, et al. Defining early mycosis fungoides. J Am Acad Dermatol 2005;53(6):1053–63.
5. Guitart J, Kennedy J, Ronan S, et al. Histologic criteria for the diagnosis of mycosis fungoides: proposal for a grading system to standardize pathology reporting. J Cutan Pathol 2001;28(4):174–83.
6. Litvinov IV, Netchiporouk E, Cordeiro B, et al. The use of transcriptional profiling to improve personalized diagnosis and management of cutaneous T-cell lymphoma (CTCL). Clin Cancer Res 2015;21(12):2820–9.
7. Litvinov IV, Tetzlaff MT, Thibault P, et al. Gene expression analysis in Cutaneous T-Cell Lymphomas (CTCL) highlights disease heterogeneity and potential diagnostic and prognostic indicators. Oncoimmunology 2017;6(5):e1306618.
8. Zhang Y, Wang Y, Yu R, et al. Molecular markers of early-stage mycosis fungoides. J Invest Dermatol 2012;132(6):1698–706.
9. Olsen E, Vonderheid E, Pimpinelli N, et al. Revisions to the staging and classification of mycosis fungoides and Sezary syndrome: a proposal of the International Society for Cutaneous Lymphomas (ISCL) and the cutaneous lymphoma task force of the European Organization of Research and Treatment of Cancer (EORTC). Blood 2007;110(6):1713–22.
10. Olsen EA, Whittaker S, Kim YH, et al. Clinical end points and response criteria in mycosis fungoides and Sezary syndrome: a consensus statement of the International Society for Cutaneous Lymphomas, the United States cutaneous lymphoma consortium, and the cutaneous lymphoma task force of the European Organisation for Research and Treatment of Cancer. J Clin Oncol 2011;29(18):2598–607.
11. Willemze R, Jaffe ES, Burg G, et al. WHO-EORTC classification for cutaneous lymphomas. Blood 2005;105(10):3768–85.
12. Ahn CS, ALSayyah A, Sangueza OP. Mycosis fungoides: an updated review of clinicopathologic variants. Am J Dermatopathol 2014;36(12):933–48 [quiz: 949–51].
13. Agar NS, Wedgeworth E, Crichton S, et al. Survival outcomes and prognostic factors in mycosis fungoides/Sezary syndrome: validation of the revised International Society for Cutaneous Lymphomas/European Organisation for Research and Treatment of Cancer staging proposal. J Clin Oncol 2010;28(31):4730–9.
14. Scarisbrick JJ, Prince HM, Vermeer MH, et al. Cutaneous lymphoma international consortium study of outcome in advanced stages of mycosis fungoides and

sezary syndrome: effect of specific prognostic markers on survival and development of a prognostic model. J Clin Oncol 2015;33(32):3766–73.

15. de Masson A, O'Malley JT, Elco CP, et al. High-throughput sequencing of the T cell receptor beta gene identifies aggressive early-stage mycosis fungoides. Sci Transl Med 2018;10(440) [pii:eaar5894].

16. Weng WK, Armstrong R, Arai S, et al. Minimal residual disease monitoring with high-throughput sequencing of T cell receptors in cutaneous T cell lymphoma. Sci Transl Med 2013;5(214):214ra171.

17. Campbell JJ, Clark RA, Watanabe R, et al. Sezary syndrome and mycosis fungoides arise from distinct T-cell subsets: a biologic rationale for their distinct clinical behaviors. Blood 2010;116(5):767–71.

18. Clark RA, Chong B, Mirchandani N, et al. The vast majority of CLA+ T cells are resident in normal skin. J Immunol 2006;176(7):4431–9.

19. Wang XN, McGovern N, Gunawan M, et al. A three-dimensional atlas of human dermal leukocytes, lymphatics, and blood vessels. J Invest Dermatol 2014; 134(4):965–74.

20. Clark RA. Skin-resident T cells: the ups and downs of on site immunity. J Invest Dermatol 2010;130(2):362–70.

21. Clark RA. Resident memory T cells in human health and disease. Sci Transl Med 2015;7(269):269rv261.

22. Watanabe R, Gehad A, Yang C, et al. Human skin is protected by four functionally and phenotypically discrete populations of resident and recirculating memory T cells. Sci Transl Med 2015;7(279):279ra239.

23. Watanabe R, Teague JE, Fisher DC, et al. Alemtuzumab therapy for leukemic cutaneous T-cell lymphoma: diffuse erythema as a positive predictor of complete remission. JAMA Dermatol 2014;150(7):776–9.

24. Clark RA, Watanabe R, Teague JE, et al. Skin effector memory T cells do not recirculate and provide immune protection in alemtuzumab-treated CTCL patients. Sci Transl Med 2012;4(117):117ra117.

25. Choi J, Goh G, Walradt T, et al. Genomic landscape of cutaneous T cell lymphoma. Nat Genet 2015;47(9):1011–9.

26. da Silva Almeida AC, Abate F, Khiabanian H, et al. The mutational landscape of cutaneous T cell lymphoma and Sezary syndrome. Nat Genet 2015;47(12): 1465–70.

27. Wang L, Ni X, Covington KR, et al. Genomic profiling of Sezary syndrome identifies alterations of key T cell signaling and differentiation genes. Nat Genet 2015;47(12):1426–34.

28. Park J, Yang J, Wenzel AT, et al. Genomic analysis of 220 CTCLs identifies a novel recurrent gain-of-function alteration in RLTPR (p.Q575E). Blood 2017;130(12): 1430–40.

29. van Doorn R, Slieker RC, Boonk SE, et al. Epigenomic analysis of sezary syndrome defines patterns of aberrant DNA methylation and identifies diagnostic markers. J Invest Dermatol 2016;136(9):1876–84.

30. Damsky WE, Choi J. Genetics of cutaneous t cell lymphoma: from bench to bedside. Curr Treat Options Oncol 2016;17(7):33.

31. Chevret E, Merlio JP. Sezary syndrome: translating genetic diversity into personalized medicine. J Invest Dermatol 2016;136(7):1319–24.

32. Qu K, Zaba LC, Satpathy AT, et al. Chromatin accessibility landscape of cutaneous T cell lymphoma and dynamic response to HDAC inhibitors. Cancer Cell 2017;32(1):27–41 e24.

33. Axelrod PI, Lorber B, Vonderheid EC. Infections complicating mycosis fungoides and Sezary syndrome. JAMA 1992;267(10):1354–8.

34. Olsen EA, Rook AH, Zic J, et al. Sezary syndrome: immunopathogenesis, literature review of therapeutic options, and recommendations for therapy by the United States Cutaneous Lymphoma Consortium (USCLC). J Am Acad Dermatol 2011;64(2):352–404.

35. Netchiporouk E, Litvinov IV, Moreau L, et al. Deregulation in STAT signaling is important for cutaneous T-cell lymphoma (CTCL) pathogenesis and cancer progression. Cell Cycle 2014;13(21):3331–5.

36. Vowels BR, Lessin SR, Cassin M, et al. Th2 cytokine mRNA expression in skin in cutaneous T-cell lymphoma. J Invest Dermatol 1994;103(5):669–73.

37. Kim EJ, Hess S, Richardson SK, et al. Immunopathogenesis and therapy of cutaneous T cell lymphoma. J Clin Invest 2005;115(4):798–812.

38. Rubio Gonzalez B, Zain J, Rosen ST, et al. Tumor microenvironment in mycosis fungoides and Sezary syndrome. Curr Opin Oncol 2016;28(1):88–96.

39. Guenova E, Watanabe R, Teague JE, et al. TH2 cytokines from malignant cells suppress TH1 responses and enforce a global TH2 bias in leukemic cutaneous T-cell lymphoma. Clin Cancer Res 2013;19(14):3755–63.

40. Tan RS, Butterworth CM, McLaughlin H, et al. Mycosis fungoides–a disease of antigen persistence. Br J Dermatol 1974;91(6):607–16.

41. Berger CL, Hanlon D, Kanada D, et al. The growth of cutaneous T-cell lymphoma is stimulated by immature dendritic cells. Blood 2002;99(8):2929–39.

42. Krejsgaard T, Willerslev-Olsen A, Lindahl LM, et al. Staphylococcal enterotoxins stimulate lymphoma-associated immune dysregulation. Blood 2014;124(5):761–70.

43. Gelfand JM, Shin DB, Neimann AL, et al. The risk of lymphoma in patients with psoriasis. J Invest Dermatol 2006;126(10):2194–201.

44. Legendre L, Barnetche T, Mazereeuw-Hautier J, et al. Risk of lymphoma in patients with atopic dermatitis and the role of topical treatment: a systematic review and meta-analysis. J Am Acad Dermatol 2015;72(6):992–1002.

45. Mirvish ED, Pomerantz RG, Geskin LJ. Infectious agents in cutaneous T-cell lymphoma. J Am Acad Dermatol 2011;64(2):423–31.

46. Mirvish JJ, Pomerantz RG, Falo LD Jr, et al. Role of infectious agents in cutaneous T-cell lymphoma: facts and controversies. Clin Dermatol 2013;31(4):423–31.

47. Anderson ME, Nagy-Szakal D, Jain K, et al. Highly sensitive virome capture sequencing technique VirCapSeq-VERT identifies partial noncoding sequences but no active viral infection in cutaneous T-cell lymphoma. J Invest Dermatol 2018;138(7):1671–3.

48. Young GR, Stoye JP, Kassiotis G. Are human endogenous retroviruses pathogenic? An approach to testing the hypothesis. Bioessays 2013;35(9):794–803.

49. Trautinger F, Eder J, Assaf C, et al. European Organisation for Research and Treatment of Cancer consensus recommendations for the treatment of mycosis fungoides/Sezary syndrome - Update 2017. Eur J Cancer 2017;77:57–74.

50. Duvic M, Hymes K, Heald P, et al. Bexarotene is effective and safe for treatment of refractory advanced-stage cutaneous T-cell lymphoma: multinational phase II-III trial results. J Clin Oncol 2001;19(9):2456–71.

51. Olsen EA, Rosen ST, Vollmer RT, et al. Interferon alfa-2a in the treatment of cutaneous T cell lymphoma. J Am Acad Dermatol 1989;20(3):395–407.

52. Whittaker SJ, Demierre MF, Kim EJ, et al. Final results from a multicenter, international, pivotal study of romidepsin in refractory cutaneous T-cell lymphoma. J Clin Oncol 2010;28(29):4485–91.

53. Zackheim HS, Kashani-Sabet M, Hwang ST. Low-dose methotrexate to treat erythrodermic cutaneous T-cell lymphoma: results in twenty-nine patients. J Am Acad Dermatol 1996;34(4):626–31.
54. Zackheim HS, Kashani-Sabet M, McMillan A. Low-dose methotrexate to treat mycosis fungoides: a retrospective study in 69 patients. J Am Acad Dermatol 2003;49(5):873–8.
55. Prince HM, Kim YH, Horwitz SM, et al. Brentuximab vedotin or physician's choice in CD30-positive cutaneous T-cell lymphoma (ALCANZA): an international, open-label, randomised, phase 3, multicentre trial. Lancet 2017;390(10094):555–66.
56. Horwitz SM, Kim YH, Foss F, et al. Identification of an active, well-tolerated dose of pralatrexate in patients with relapsed or refractory cutaneous T-cell lymphoma. Blood 2012;119(18):4115–22.
57. Quereux G, Marques S, Nguyen JM, et al. Prospective multicenter study of pegylated liposomal doxorubicin treatment in patients with advanced or refractory mycosis fungoides or Sezary syndrome. Arch Dermatol 2008;144(6):727–33.
58. Zinzani PL, Baliva G, Magagnoli M, et al. Gemcitabine treatment in pretreated cutaneous T-cell lymphoma: experience in 44 patients. J Clin Oncol 2000; 18(13):2603–6.
59. Zinzani PL, Musuraca G, Tani M, et al. Phase II trial of proteasome inhibitor bortezomib in patients with relapsed or refractory cutaneous T-cell lymphoma. J Clin Oncol 2007;25(27):4293–7.
60. Zinzani PL, Venturini F, Stefoni V, et al. Gemcitabine as single agent in pretreated T-cell lymphoma patients: evaluation of the long-term outcome. Ann Oncol 2010; 21(4):860–3.
61. Khodadoust M, RA, Porcu P. Pembrolizumab for treatment of relapsed/refrectory mycosis fungoides and Sezary Syndrome: clinical efficacy in a CITN multicenter phase 2 study [abstact]. Blood 2016;125(Abstract 181).
62. Hanel W, Briski R, Ross CW, et al. A retrospective comparative outcome analysis following systemic therapy in Mycosis fungoides and Sezary syndrome. Am J Hematol 2016;91(12):E491–5.
63. Wilcox RA. Cutaneous T-cell lymphoma: 2017 update on diagnosis, risk-stratification, and management. Am J Hematol 2017;92(10):1085–102.
64. Hughes CF, Khot A, McCormack C, et al. Lack of durable disease control with chemotherapy for mycosis fungoides and Sezary syndrome: a comparative study of systemic therapy. Blood 2015;125(1):71–81.
65. Duarte RF, Boumendll A, Onida F, et al. Long-term outcome of allogeneic hematopoietic cell transplantation for patients with mycosis fungoides and Sezary syndrome: a European society for blood and marrow transplantation lymphoma working party extended analysis. J Clin Oncol 2014;32(29):3347–8.
66. Weng WKAR, Arai S, Johnston L, et al. Non-myeloablative allogeneic transplantation resulting in clinical and molecular remission with low Non-Relapse Mortality (NRM) in patients with advanced stage Mycosis Fungoides (MF) and Sézary Syndrome (SS). Blood 2014;124:2544.

A Review of Primary Cutaneous CD30⁺ Lymphoproliferative Disorders

Cynthia Chen, BSa, Yuhan D. Gu, BSa, Larisa J. Geskin, MDb,*

KEYWORDS

- CD30 • Lymphoproliferative • LyP • pcALCL • CTCL

KEY POINTS

- Primary cutaneous CD30⁺ lymphoproliferative diseases (pcCD30⁺ LPDs) have varied histologic and phenotypic characteristics, although all have favorable prognoses.
- The 2 major forms of pcCD30⁺ LPDs are lymphomatoid papulosis, which presents with self-resolving crops of small papules or nodules, and primary cutaneous anaplastic large cell lymphoma, which presents with large fixed nodules or tumors.
- Secondary malignancies should be considered as part of the initial evaluation, and patients diagnosed with pcCD30⁺ LPDs should have ongoing surveillance.

INTRODUCTION

Primary cutaneous CD30-positive lymphoproliferative disorders (pcCD30⁺ LPD) are a heterogeneous group comprising lymphomatoid papulosis (LyP), primary cutaneous anaplastic large cell lymphoma (pcALCL), transformed mycosis fungoides (MF), and borderline lesions. It is the second most common form of cutaneous T-cell lymphomas (CTCL), accounting for up to 30% of patients.[1] Although LyP and pcALCL are distinct clinical entities, they are now thought of as part of the same spectrum of disease with overlapping features. Some patients can have both disorders, leading to the designation of such cases as borderline or indeterminate until the clinical course points toward a specific diagnosis.[1] CD30⁺ transformed MF is a specific secondary CD30⁺ condition, which appears in the context of preexisting MF and carries a particularly poor prognosis. The authors focus this review on the pcCD30⁺ LPDs.

The hallmark of both LyP and pcALCL is the presence of atypical T lymphocytes that express CD30 on a lesional skin biopsy. CD30, also known as Ki-1 antigen, is a

Disclosure Statement: All authors have no disclosures.
a Columbia University Vagelos College of Physicians and Surgeons, 161 Fort Washington Avenue, New York, NY 10032, USA; b Department of Dermatology, Columbia University, 161 Fort Washington Avenue, New York, NY 10032, USA
* Corresponding author.
E-mail address: ljg2145@cumc.columbia.edu

Hematol Oncol Clin N Am 33 (2019) 121–134
https://doi.org/10.1016/j.hoc.2018.08.003   hemonc.theclinics.com

transmembrane receptor and a member of the tumor necrosis factor superfamily, first identified in 1982 as a surface marker for select Hodgkin lymphoma (HL) cell lines.[2] Under physiologic conditions, CD30 is expressed by a subset of activated T and B lymphocytes, and its interaction with CD30 ligand (CD30L) is thought to mediate T-cell–driven immune response to antigen stimulation through downstream signaling pathways, including NF-kB and MAPK/ERK.[3] CD30 is also overexpressed in HL, systemic ALCL, and some B-cell lymphomas, and it may be overexpressed in MF and in inflammatory conditions like atopic dermatitis, rheumatoid arthritis, and systemic lupus erythematosus.[4,5] The role of CD30 in lymphomagenesis has not been worked out, but studies thus far demonstrate pleiotropic effects of CD30 stimulation in different lymphomas with regards to proliferation, apoptosis, and cell-cycle regulation.[6,7]

CD30[+] infiltrates can be found in a wide range of cutaneous disorders as shown in **Fig. 1**, broadly categorized as either neoplastic or reactive/benign. The workup for these patients is delineated in **Fig. 2** and begins with an adequate biopsy of the suspicious lesions for histologic studies, immunophenotyping, and polymerase chain reaction for clonal T-cell receptor (TCR) rearrangement. A low threshold for further workup to exclude malignant lymphoma is recommended, as appropriate. This review describes the key features of the 2 types of CD30[+] LPD, LyP and pcALCL, focusing on their clinical presentations, histopathology, management, and treatment modalities.

LYMPHOMATOID PAPULOSIS
Overview and Pathogenesis

The first case of LyP was reported by Dr Warren L. Macauley in 1968 as a clinically benign but histologically malignant disorder of unknown cause that presents with "rhythmic paradoxic eruptions."[8] It was not until almost 20 years later that biopsies from patients with LyP demonstrated large atypical cells that stained CD30 positive,[9] giving rise to the current classification of LyP as a CD30[+] LPD on the same spectrum as other CTCLs.[1] Although largely a benign disease, up to 60% of cases occur in conjunction with malignant lymphomas, and some argue that LyP should be considered and managed as a low-grade malignancy.

The pathogenesis of LyP is unknown, but studies have implicated genetic abnormalities in CD30 transcription as well as aberrant interactions between CD30 and its ligand CD30L in the development and natural history of LyP.[10,11] A viral cause has also been postulated given recently published cases of LyP with clonal integration of human T-lymphotropic virus 1 and with infiltration of lesional dermal endothelial cells by hepatitis E virus.[12,13] Nevertheless, many other studies have shown no association between LyP and other exogenous viruses, including retro, herpes, and poxviruses.[14–16] LyP has also been theorized to be related to chronic inflammatory stimulation of the skin, oftentimes a result of skin injury or infections, leading to the recruitment of abnormal CD30[+] cells seen on biopsy. This model of chronic inflammation and tumorigenesis has been well established in the pathogenesis of a wide range of cancers and more recently in MF[17–19] and is supported by reports of LyP developing in the area previously exposed to radiotherapy for breast carcinoma[20] and in patients with MF who were being treated with topical nitrogen mustard gel (Geskin LJ, unpublished observation, 2018).

Clinical Presentation and Epidemiology

LyP typically presents as recurrent polymorphous erythematous or violaceous papulonodules (**Fig. 3**). Lesions are predominantly on the trunk and extremities and may

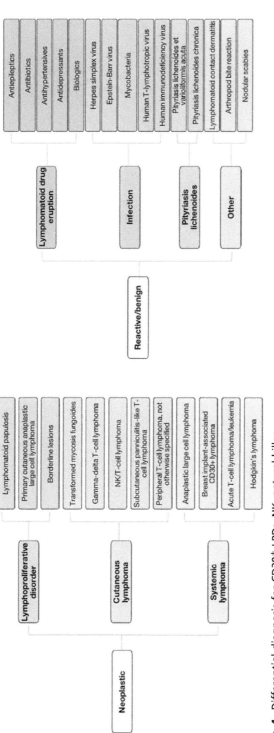

Fig. 1. Differential diagnosis for CD30⁺ LPDs. NK, natural killer.

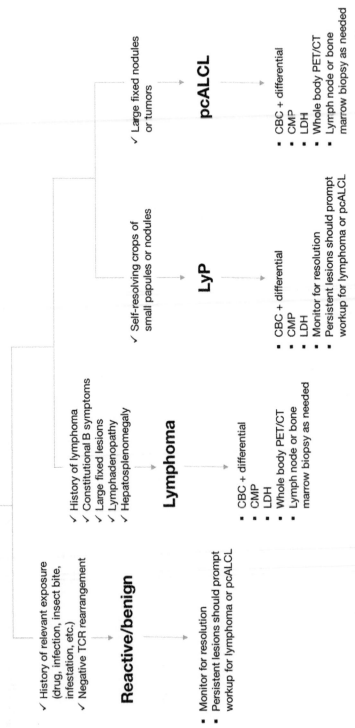

Fig. 2. Workup algorithm for histologic finding of a CD30+ infiltrate on skin biopsy. CBC, complete blood count; CMP, complete metabolic profile; LDH, lactate dehydrogenase.

develop ulceration especially in the angioinvasive subtype. Other presentations that have been reported in the literature include pustular,[21] follicular,[22] mucosal,[23] regional,[24] and persistent agminated (papules within MF-like patch),[25] among other variants. Lesions can be pruritic, tender, or asymptomatic, and importantly, LyP patients usually do not have constitutional symptoms unlike those with an associated malignant lymphoma. The key feature of LyP that helps distinguish it from other CD30⁺ LPDs is its waxing and waning clinical course, with lesions regressing spontaneously within 4 to 8 weeks.[4] Disease course and duration are highly variable, with some patients experiencing a single outbreak, whereas others develop frequent lesions for decades. LyP is the most common form of CD30⁺ LPDs and presents most often in adults with no clear predilection for a certain gender or ethnicity. Pediatric cases are rare but have been reported and shown to have a similar presentation as adult cases, including the increased risk of malignancy.[26]

Histopathology

As of 2016, there are 6 World Health Organization–recognized histologic subtypes of LyP as summarized in **Table 1**, with common features including the presence of atypical CD30⁺ lymphocytes in the dermis with varying degrees of neutrophilic or eosinophilic infiltration.[27] Several additional variants have also been proposed in recent years, including folliculotropic (type F),[22] granulomatous eccinotropic,[28] intralymphatic,[29] and spindle cell variants.[30] Of all these subtypes, type A is the most common histopathologic manifestation found in 75% of all LyP biopsies. Notably, the infiltrating lymphocytes in type B display a cerebriform nuclei and can be CD30-negative

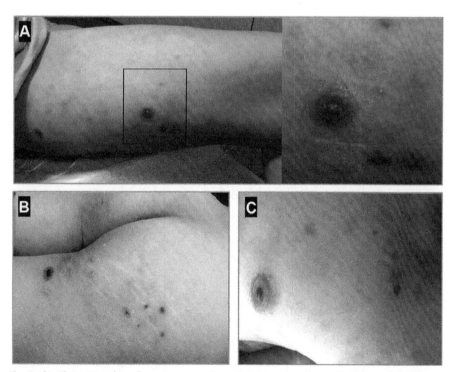

Fig. 3. (*A–C*) Scattered erythematous papulonodules representing LyP lesions of 3 different patients.

Table 1
Histologic subtypes of LyP

Type	Histology	Immunophenotype	Differential Diagnoses
A	Wedge-shaped infiltrate of large lymphocytes, numerous inflammatory cells	$CD4^+$ $CD8^-$ $CD30^+$	• HL • Transformed MF
B	Epidermotropic infiltrate of small lymphocytes with cerebriform nuclei	$CD4^+$ $CD8^-$ $CD30^{+/-}$	• MF/Sezary
C	Dense dermal infiltrate of large lymphocytes, few inflammatory cells	$CD4^+$ $CD8^-$ $CD30^+$	• pcALCL • Transformed MF
D	Pagetoid/epidermotropic infiltrate of small lymphocytes	$CD4^-$ $CD8^+$ $CD30^+$	• $CD8^+$ cytotoxic lymphoma • Pagetoid reticulosis
E	Dermal angiocentric infiltrates of medium lymphocytes, fibrinous vasculitis, and/or thrombi	$CD4^-$ $CD8^+$ $CD30^+$	• Extranodal NK/T-cell lymphoma • Gamma/delta lymphoma • Angioinvasive pcALCL
6p25.3	Pagetoid/epidermotropic infiltrate of small lymphocytes with cerebriform nuclei, dense dermal infiltrate of large atypical lymphocytes	$CD4^-$ $CD8^-$ $CD30^+$	• Pagetoid reticulosis • MF/Sezary

Data from Swerdlow SH, Campo E, Pileri SA, et al. The 2016 revision of the World Health Organization classification of lymphoid neoplasms. Blood 2016;127(20):2375–90.

mimicking MF or Sezary syndrome, and type D and E infiltrates stain CD8-positive and are often mistaken for more aggressive lymphomas. In addition, clonal T-cell populations have been detected in most skin biopsies positive for LyP, and T-cell clones have even been reported in the peripheral blood of LyP patients, although it is controversial whether those in the blood are reactive rather than derived from the same origin as those in the skin.[31–33]

Despite the significant variations between LyP lesions under the microscope, all subtypes present with a similar clinical picture, except for type E, which is distinguished by rapidly evolving papulonodules that ulcerate and form large escharlike necrotic lesions.[34] Moreover, studies have thus far shown no overall prognostic differences between the different subtypes, although a recent retrospective study showed that types B and C are associated with an increased risk of subsequently developing lymphoma.[35] There is also overlap between these subtypes because patients can present with concurrent lesions of different subtypes and with individual lesions that fit the criteria for multiple subtypes.

Diagnosis and Management

LyP is diagnosed based on a combination of clinical features and histopathologic and immunohistochemical findings. Current recommendations include obtaining a complete blood cell count with differential, blood chemistry, and lactate dehydrogenase for all patients.[36] If there is any suspicion for malignancy, for example, presence of B symptoms, enlarged lymph nodes, large lesions that do not spontaneously regress, or abnormal blood work, further laboratory or radiological studies or bone marrow biopsy may be needed. Additional attention should be paid to the patients with prior history of lymphoma.

LyP lesions usually resolve on their own with no intervention, and thus observation is an acceptable approach for patients with few lesions that are relatively asymptomatic. If necessary, symptomatic management for localized disease can be provided with topical corticosteroids, which may hasten recovery but do not prevent reoccurrence. Symptomatic patients may also benefit from phototherapy with either psoralen–UV-A or UV-B, with studies showing not only faster clearance but also less frequent relapses while on maintenance therapy.[36] Nevertheless, the risks of developing melanoma and nonmelanoma skin cancers should be weighed in the decision to initiate phototherapy for patients with LyP.

For patients with generalized lesions and a high symptom burden, low-dose methotrexate is the recommended first-line treatment based on several observational studies that demonstrate response rates, both complete and partial, of greater than 80%.[37–39] The difficulty with using methotrexate is the need for long-term maintenance therapy in most patients, compounded with serious drug side effects, including hepatotoxicity, pulmonary fibrosis, and myelosuppression. Recently, another systemic treatment, brentuximab vedotin, a monoclonal antibody-drug conjugate against the CD30 receptor, which was approved for relapsed non-HL and systemic ALCL, has been shown in a phase 2 clinical trial to induce a 100% response rate in patients with LyP and pcALCL, with an average response duration of 26 weeks.[40] Unfortunately, its long-term toxicity, such as irreversible neuropathy, limits its prolonged use. Finally, there are also reports of successful treatment of LyP with bexarotene,[41,42] topical chemotherapy (nitrogen mustard or carmustine),[43] and photodynamic therapy.[44]

Prognosis and Associated Lymphomas

Overall, LyP is a chronic indolent disease with an excellent prognosis. A retrospective cohort analysis found that no patients with LyP died of the disease with an overall survival rate of 92% at 10 years.[45] Nevertheless, LyP lies on the same spectrum as pcALCL and other malignant CTCLs, and up to 60% of cases occur in conjunction with malignant lymphomas that may be develop before, after, or at the same time as the diagnosis of LyP with highly variable time courses. Large retrospective cohort studies have shown that the most common associated malignancy is MF, constituting more than 50% of patients, followed by ALCL and HL. Risk factors for development of lymphoma include male gender and histologic subtypes B and C, all found to have greater than 2.5 times increased risk.[35,46] Interestingly, LyP disease severity had no impact on risk, and furthermore, presence of a clonal TCR gene rearrangement was not found to increase risk of a secondary lymphoma, despite studies showing that the atypical lymphoid cells seen in LyP lesions can exhibit clonal TCR rearrangements that are often identical to those in concurrent lymphomas.[35,47,48]

It is not possible to predict which patients will progress to lymphoma, and importantly, no treatment of LyP has been found to prevent the development of an associated lymphoma or decrease risk. Thus, all patients must be counseled and closely monitored with regards to the development of nonregressing erythematous patches, plaques, or tumors or new enlarged lymph nodes, in addition to any constitutional symptoms.

PRIMARY CUTANEOUS ANAPLASTIC LARGE CELL LYMPHOMA
Overview

Anaplastic large cell lymphoma, a subset of peripheral T-cell lymphoma, was first described in 1985 as a lymphoid malignancy with strong CD30 expression that can present clinically with systemic or with localized cutaneous disease.[49] Because of genetic, immunohistological, and clinical differences, systemic and primary cutaneous ALCL have been recognized as distinct entities, with the latter having more favorable prognosis despite having rapidly growing lesions and CD30 tumor cells demonstrating highly atypical cytomorphology.[50]

Clinical Presentation and Epidemiology

Most patients with pcALCL present with individual or grouped red/brown cutaneous nodules that grow rapidly over the course of weeks to months (**Fig. 4**). These lesions have a tendency to ulcerate and have a proclivity for the head and neck region and the extremities.[51] Although most patients have fixed lesions that do not resolve without treatment, up to 40% can in fact experience spontaneous complete or partial

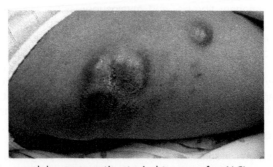

Fig. 4. Erythematous nodules representing typical tumors of pcALCL.

regression of pcALCL lesions.[4] Nevertheless, relapses are common, with 39% of patients developing recurrent skin lesions and 13% developing extracutaneous involvement.[45] Most patients present with a solitary lesion, and approximately one-fifth present with multifocal disease involving different anatomic sites. One specific subset of patients who develop multiple lower extremity lesions, termed "extensive limb disease," has a more aggressive clinical course and overall poorer prognosis.[52] Unlike systemic ALCL, patients with pcALCL generally do not report systemic B symptoms and patients who do should be further evaluated for systemic disease. Although the exact incidence is not known, pcALCL is a rare disease and is the second most common form of CD30+ LPDs, estimated to account for approximately 40% of such patients.[4] The median age of diagnosis of pcALCL is around 60 years old with a slight male predominance.[53]

Histopathology

pcALCL skin biopsies are characterized by dense nodular or diffuse infiltrates of large lymphoid cells in the dermis, usually with no epidermal involvement. The large infiltrating anaplastic lymphocytes have irregular, often horseshoe-shaped nuclei, prominent eosinophilic nucleoli, and abundant cytoplasm.[36] In approximately one-quarter of cases, however, pcALCL can have an immunoblastic or nonanaplastic pleomorphic morphology.[54] In these cases, a heterogeneous inflammatory infiltrate including neutrophils and eosinophils may be present.

By definition, CD30 must be expressed by at least 75% of the aberrant lymphocytes. These tumor cells resemble activated T cells, and most cases show CD4 expression with variable loss of CD2, CD3, and CD5.[1] There is significant phenotypic variability in CD4 and CD8 expression, in contrast to previous reports, which hypothesized a CD4+/CD8- predominance.[55] The translocation t(2;5)(p23;q35) of anaplastic lymphoma kinase (ALK) and nucleophosmin is almost always negative in PCALCL, although recent reports have described rare cases of ALK-positive primary cutaneous disease.[56] It is important to note that ALK-negativity does not rule out systemic ALCL given that it is negative in approximately 50% of systemic ALCL cases. Most pcALCL demonstrate clonal rearrangement of the TCR, present in 90% of cases.[57] Chromosomal rearrangements of the DUSP22-IRF4 locus on 6p25.3 have also been frequently detected.[58]

Workup and Staging

Whenever a diagnosis of pcALCL is suspected based on clinicopathologic features, it is crucial to exclude a cutaneous manifestation of a systemic lymphoma with not only assessment of constitutional symptoms and basic laboratory studies as in the workup of LyP but also radiologic studies, preferably whole body PET combined with computed tomography (PET-CT).[36] Lymph node biopsies should be performed to rule out nodal lymphoma if lymphadenopathy is present on examination or avid nodes are seen on PET-CT. However, bone marrow biopsy is no longer recommended for patients with pcALCL unless widespread tumors or abnormal laboratory or radiologic results strongly suggest extracutaneous disease.[59]

Staging of pcALCL, as well as LyP, should be performed according to a European Organisation for Research and Treatment of Cancer (EORTC) and International Society for Cutaneous Lymphomas (ISCL) proposed TMN classification system for all primary cutaneous lymphomas other than MF and Sezary syndrome.[60] Although this system was largely intended to serve as a unified way to document extent of disease, recent studies have shown that it can also be a helpful prognostic guide.[61]

Management and Prognosis

Patients presenting with solitary or localized lesions, regardless of whether they represent initial or relapsed disease, should be treated with complete surgical excision or radiotherapy.[36] Both have been found to be well tolerated and to induce complete remission in almost 100% of patients treated with either modality.[45] Skin-limited recurrence rates however occurred in around 40% of all patients with no increase in disease-free duration after combined excision and radiotherapy.[45,62,63] Patients with regional lymph node involvement are treated with radiation to both the cutaneous lesions and the affected nodes.

Multifocal pcALCL, as well as frequent recurrent lesions, is treated with systemic therapy, similar to that used for generalized and highly symptomatic LyP. Current guidelines recommend methotrexate as the first-line agent with one retrospective study showing 77% response rates within 4 weeks, although long-term maintenance therapy is needed to prevent recurrence.[37] Bexarotene may be used as an alternative treatment for patients who cannot tolerate or have disease progression on methotrexate, although evidence for this is based mainly from case reports.[64,65] Recently, brentuximab vedotin has also emerged as a treatment option for multifocal pcALCL, with a phase 3 trial showing superior response rates, progression-free survival, and symptomatic relief compared with either methotrexate or bexarotene.[66] Finally, there is anecdotal evidence for the use of interferon, especially in combination with bexarotene,[67,68] thalidomide,[69] gemcitabine,[70] and etoposide,[71] in multifocal pcALCL. Importantly, multiagent chemotherapy, which had previously been used as first-line therapy for advanced pcALCL, is no longer recommended given high relapse rates of up to 70% and an excellent overall prognosis. It is now reserved only for extracutaneous spread.[4,36]

Patients with pcALCL can generally expect an indolent disease course and excellent prognoses, with disease-specific survival rates of 85% to 90% at 10 years. Factors associated with worse prognosis include more extensive or higher stage (T2 or T3) disease, leg involvement, immunosuppression, and extracutaneous spread.[45,52,61,72] Interestingly, skin-restricted recurrences and locoregional node involvement do not affect prognosis.[4,61]

SUMMARY

pcCD30+ LPD comprise a range of diseases (LyP, pcALCL, and borderline lesions) with broad histologic and phenotypical characteristics, although they all share the common feature of a favorable prognosis notwithstanding histology, suggestive of a high-grade lymphoma. Given their cytomorphologic similarities, accurate diagnosis and workup require differentiating these distinct entities based on clinical presentation, lesional progression, and clinicopathologic correlation in order to best use novel biologic therapies and avoid aggressive overtreatment. Moreover, although CD30+ LPD has a favorable prognosis, secondary malignancies should be considered as part of the initial evaluation and patients should have ongoing surveillance.

REFERENCES

1. Willemze R, Jaffe ES, Burg G, et al. WHO-EORTC classification for cutaneous lymphomas. Blood 2005;105(10):3768–85.
2. Stein H, Gerdes J, Schwab U, et al. Identification of Hodgkin and Sternberg-reed cells as a unique cell type derived from a newly-detected small-cell population. Int J Cancer 1982;30(4):445–59.

3. Horie R, Watanabe T. CD30: expression and function in health and disease. Semin Immunol 1998;10(6):457–70.
4. Bekkenk MW, Geelen FA, van Voorst Vader PC, et al. Primary and secondary cutaneous CD30(+) lymphoproliferative disorders: a report from the Dutch Cutaneous Lymphoma Group on the long-term follow-up data of 219 patients and guidelines for diagnosis and treatment. Blood 2000;95(12):3653–61.
5. Werner B, Massone C, Kerl H, et al. Large CD30-positive cells in benign, atypical lymphoid infiltrates of the skin. J Cutan Pathol 2008;35(12):1100–7.
6. Gruss HJ, Boiani N, Williams DE, et al. Pleiotropic effects of the CD30 ligand on CD30-expressing cells and lymphoma cell lines. Blood 1994;83(8):2045–56.
7. Kadin ME, Levi E, Kempf W. Progression of lymphomatoid papulosis to systemic lymphoma is associated with escape from growth inhibition by transforming growth factor-beta and CD30 ligand. Ann N Y Acad Sci 2001;941:59–68.
8. Macaulay WL. Lymphomatoid papulosis. A continuing self-healing eruption, clinically benign–histologically malignant. Arch Dermatol 1968;97(1):23–30.
9. Kadin M, Nasu K, Sako D, et al. Lymphomatoid papulosis. A cutaneous proliferation of activated helper T cells expressing Hodgkin's disease-associated antigens. Am J Pathol 1985;119(2):315–25.
10. Mori M, Manuelli C, Pimpinelli N, et al. CD30-CD30 ligand interaction in primary cutaneous CD30(+) T-cell lymphomas: a clue to the pathophysiology of clinical regression. Blood 1999;94(9):3077–83.
11. Franchina M, Kadin ME, Abraham LJ. Polymorphism of the CD30 promoter microsatellite repressive element is associated with development of primary cutaneous lymphoproliferative disorders. Cancer Epidemiol Biomarkers Prev 2005;14(5): 1322–5.
12. Namba H, Hamada T, Iwatsuki K. Human T-cell leukemia virus type 1-positive lymphomatoid papulosis. Eur J Dermatol 2016;26(2):194–5.
13. Mallet V, Bruneau J, Zuber J, et al. Hepatitis E virus-induced primary cutaneous CD30(+) T cell lymphoproliferative disorder. J Hepatol 2017;67(6):1334–9.
14. Kempf W, Kadin ME, Dvorak AM, et al. Endogenous retroviral elements, but not exogenous retroviruses, are detected in CD30-positive lymphoproliferative disorders of the skin. Carcinogenesis 2003;24(2):301–6.
15. Kempf W, Kadin ME, Kutzner H, et al. Lymphomatoid papulosis and human herpesviruses–A PCR-based evaluation for the presence of human herpesvirus 6, 7 and 8 related herpesviruses. J Cutan Pathol 2001;28(1):29–33.
16. Fernandez KH, Bream M, Ali MA, et al. Investigation of molluscum contagiosum virus, orf and other parapoxviruses in lymphomatoid papulosis. J Am Acad Dermatol 2013;68(6):1046–7.
17. Grivennikov SI, Greten FR, Karin M. Immunity, inflammation, and cancer. Cell 2010;140(6):883–99.
18. Lowe DB, Storkus WJ. Chronic inflammation and immunologic-based constraints in malignant disease. Immunotherapy 2011;3(10):1265–74.
19. Krejsgaard T, Lindahl LM, Mongan NP, et al. Malignant inflammation in cutaneous T-cell lymphoma-a hostile takeover. Semin Immunopathol 2017;39(3):269–82.
20. Haro R, Juarez A, Diaz JL, et al. Regional lymphomatoid papulosis of the breast restricted to an area of prior radiotherapy. Cutis 2016;97(5):E15–9.
21. Barnadas MA, Lopez D, Pujol RM, et al. Pustular lymphomatoid papulosis in childhood. J Am Acad Dermatol 1992;27(4):627–8.
22. Kempf W, Kazakov DV, Baumgartner HP, et al. Follicular lymphomatoid papulosis revisited: a study of 11 cases, with new histopathological findings. J Am Acad Dermatol 2013;68(5):809–16.

23. Pujol RM, Muret MP, Bergua P, et al. Oral involvement in lymphomatoid papulosis. Report of two cases and review of the literature. Dermatology 2005;210(1):53–7.
24. Scarisbrick JJ, Evans AV, Woolford AJ, et al. Regional lymphomatoid papulosis: a report of four cases. Br J Dermatol 1999;141(6):1125–8.
25. Heald P, Subtil A, Breneman D, et al. Persistent agmination of lymphomatoid papulosis: an equivalent of limited plaque mycosis fungoides type of cutaneous T-cell lymphoma. J Am Acad Dermatol 2007;57(6):1005–11.
26. Nijsten T, Curiel-Lewandrowski C, Kadin ME. Lymphomatoid papulosis in children: a retrospective cohort study of 35 cases. Arch Dermatol 2004;140(3): 306–12.
27. Swerdlow SH, Campo E, Pileri SA, et al. The 2016 revision of the World Health Organization classification of lymphoid neoplasms. Blood 2016;127(20):2375–90.
28. Crowson AN, Baschinsky DY, Kovatich A, et al. Granulomatous eccrinotropic lymphomatoid papulosis. Am J Clin Pathol 2003;119(5):731–9.
29. Ferrara G, Ena L, Cota C, et al. Intralymphatic spread is a common finding in cutaneous CD30+ lymphoproliferative disorders. Am J Surg Pathol 2015; 39(11):1511–7.
30. Martires KJ, Cohen BE, Cassarino DS. CD30+ lymphoproliferative disorder with spindle-cell morphology. J Cutan Pathol 2016;43(11):1041–4.
31. Steinhoff M, Hummel M, Anagnostopoulos I, et al. Single-cell analysis of CD30+ cells in lymphomatoid papulosis demonstrates a common clonal T-cell origin. Blood 2002;100(2):578–84.
32. Schultz JC, Granados S, Vonderheid EC, et al. T-cell clonality of peripheral blood lymphocytes in patients with lymphomatoid papulosis. J Am Acad Dermatol 2005;53(1):152–5.
33. Humme D, Lukowsky A, Steinhoff M, et al. Dominance of nonmalignant T-cell clones and distortion of the TCR repertoire in the peripheral blood of patients with cutaneous CD30+ lymphoproliferative disorders. J Invest Dermatol 2009; 129(1):89–98.
34. Kempf W, Kazakov DV, Scharer L, et al. Angioinvasive lymphomatoid papulosis: a new variant simulating aggressive lymphomas. Am J Surg Pathol 2013;37(1): 1–13.
35. Wieser I, Oh CW, Talpur R, et al. Lymphomatoid papulosis: treatment response and associated lymphomas in a study of 180 patients. J Am Acad Dermatol 2016;74(1):59–67.
36. Kempf W, Pfaltz K, Vermeer MH, et al. EORTC, ISCL, and USCLC consensus recommendations for the treatment of primary cutaneous CD30-positive lymphoproliferative disorders: lymphomatoid papulosis and primary cutaneous anaplastic large-cell lymphoma. Blood 2011;118(15):4024–35.
37. Vonderheid EC, Sajjadian A, Kadin ME. Methotrexate is effective therapy for lymphomatoid papulosis and other primary cutaneous CD30-positive lymphoproliferative disorders. J Am Acad Dermatol 1996;34(3):470–81.
38. Bruijn MS, Horvath B, van Voorst Vader PC, et al. Recommendations for treatment of lymphomatoid papulosis with methotrexate: a report from the Dutch Cutaneous Lymphoma Group. Br J Dermatol 2015;173(5):1319–22.
39. Newland KM, McCormack CJ, Twigger R, et al. The efficacy of methotrexate for lymphomatoid papulosis. J Am Acad Dermatol 2015;72(6):1088–90.
40. Duvic M, Tetzlaff MT, Gangar P, et al. Results of a phase II trial of brentuximab vedotin for CD30+ cutaneous T-cell lymphoma and lymphomatoid papulosis. J Clin Oncol 2015;33(32):3759–65.

41. Krathen RA, Ward S, Duvic M. Bexarotene is a new treatment option for lympho-matoid papulosis. Dermatology 2003;206(2):142–7.
42. Fujimura T, Furudate S, Tanita K, et al. Successful control of phototherapy-resistant lymphomatoid papulosis with oral bexarotene. J Dermatol 2018;45(2): e37–8.
43. Zackheim HS, Epstein EH Jr, Crain WR. Topical carmustine therapy for lympho-matoid papulosis. Arch Dermatol 1985;121(11):1410–4.
44. Rodrigues M, McCormack C, Yap LM, et al. Successful treatment of lymphoma-toid papulosis with photodynamic therapy. Australas J Dermatol 2009;50(2): 129–32.
45. Liu HL, Hoppe RT, Kohler S, et al. CD30+ cutaneous lymphoproliferative disor-ders: the Stanford experience in lymphomatoid papulosis and primary cutaneous anaplastic large cell lymphoma. J Am Acad Dermatol 2003;49(6):1049–58.
46. Kunishige JH, McDonald H, Alvarez G, et al. Lymphomatoid papulosis and asso-ciated lymphomas: a retrospective case series of 84 patients. Clin Exp Dermatol 2009;34(5):576–81.
47. Davis TH, Morton CC, Miller-Cassman R, et al. Hodgkin's disease, lymphomatoid papulosis, and cutaneous T-cell lymphoma derived from a common T-cell clone. N Engl J Med 1992;326(17):1115–22.
48. Zackheim HS, Jones C, Leboit PE, et al. Lymphomatoid papulosis associated with mycosis fungoides: a study of 21 patients including analyses for clonality. J Am Acad Dermatol 2003;49(4):620–3.
49. Stein H, Mason DY, Gerdes J, et al. The expression of the Hodgkin's disease associated antigen Ki-1 in reactive and neoplastic lymphoid tissue: evidence that Reed-Sternberg cells and histiocytic malignancies are derived from acti-vated lymphoid cells. Blood 1985;66(4):848–58.
50. Fornari A, Piva R, Chiarle R, et al. Anaplastic large cell lymphoma: one or more entities among T-cell lymphoma? Hematol Oncol 2009;27(4):161–70.
51. Kadin ME, Carpenter C. Systemic and primary cutaneous anaplastic large cell lymphomas. Semin Hematol 2003;40(3):244–56.
52. Woo DK, Jones CR, Vanoli-Storz MN, et al. Prognostic factors in primary cuta-neous anaplastic large cell lymphoma: characterization of clinical subset with worse outcome. Arch Dermatol 2009;145(6):667–74.
53. Booken N, Goerdt S, Klemke CD. Clinical spectrum of primary cutaneous CD30-positive anaplastic large cell lymphoma: an analysis of the Mannheim Cutaneous Lymphoma Registry. J Dtsch Dermatol Ges 2012;10(5):331–9.
54. Burg G, Kempf W, Kazakov DV, et al. Pyogenic lymphoma of the skin: a peculiar variant of primary cutaneous neutrophil-rich CD30+ anaplastic large-cell lym-phoma. Clinicopathological study of four cases and review of the literature. Br J Dermatol 2003;148(3):580–6.
55. Massone C, El-Shabrawi-Caelen L, Kerl H, et al. The morphologic spectrum of primary cutaneous anaplastic large T-cell lymphoma: a histopathologic study on 66 biopsy specimens from 47 patients with report of rare variants. J Cutan Pathol 2008;35(1):46–53.
56. Oschlies I, Lisfeld J, Lamant L, et al. ALK-positive anaplastic large cell lymphoma limited to the skin: clinical, histopathological and molecular analysis of 6 pediatric cases. A report from the ALCL99 study. Haematologica 2013;98(1):50–6.
57. Macgrogan G, Vergier B, Dubus P, et al. CD30-positive cutaneous large cell lym-phomas. A comparative study of clinicopathologic and molecular features of 16 cases. Am J Clin Pathol 1996;105(4):440–50.

58. Pham-Ledard A, Prochazkova-Carlotti M, Laharanne E, et al. IRF4 gene rearrangements define a subgroup of CD30-positive cutaneous T-cell lymphoma: a study of 54 cases. J Invest Dermatol 2010;130(3):816–25.
59. Benner MF, Willemze R. Bone marrow examination has limited value in the staging of patients with an anaplastic large cell lymphoma first presenting in the skin. Retrospective analysis of 107 patients. Br J Dermatol 2008;159(5):1148–51.
60. Kim YH, Willemze R, Pimpinelli N, et al. TNM classification system for primary cutaneous lymphomas other than mycosis fungoides and Sezary syndrome: a proposal of the International Society for Cutaneous Lymphomas (ISCL) and the Cutaneous Lymphoma Task Force of the European Organization of Research and Treatment of Cancer (EORTC). Blood 2007;110(2):479–84.
61. Benner MF, Willemze R. Applicability and prognostic value of the new TNM classification system in 135 patients with primary cutaneous anaplastic large cell lymphoma. Arch Dermatol 2009;145(12):1399–404.
62. Beljaards RC, Kaudewitz P, Berti E, et al. Primary cutaneous CD30-positive large cell lymphoma: definition of a new type of cutaneous lymphoma with a favorable prognosis. A European Multicenter Study of 47 patients. Cancer 1993;71(6):2097–104.
63. Paulli M, Berti E, Rosso R, et al. CD30/Ki-1-positive lymphoproliferative disorders of the skin–clinicopathologic correlation and statistical analysis of 86 cases: a multicentric study from the European Organization for Research and Treatment of Cancer Cutaneous Lymphoma Project Group. J Clin Oncol 1995;13(6):1343–54.
64. Sheehy O, Catherwood M, Pettengell R, et al. Sustained response of primary cutaneous CD30 positive anaplastic large cell lymphoma to bexarotene and photopheresis. Leuk Lymphoma 2009;50(8):1389–91.
65. Oliveira A, Fernandes I, Alves R, et al. Primary cutaneous CD30 positive anaplastic large cell lymphoma–report of a case treated with bexarotene. Leuk Res 2011;35(11):e190–2.
66. Prince HM, Kim YH, Horwitz SM, et al. Brentuximab vedotin or physician's choice in CD30-positive cutaneous T-cell lymphoma (ALCANZA): an international, open-label, randomised, phase 3, multicentre trial. Lancet 2017;390(10094):555–66.
67. French LE, Shapiro M, Junkins-Hopkins JM, et al. Regression of multifocal, skin-restricted, CD30-positive large T-cell lymphoma with interferon alfa and bexarotene therapy. J Am Acad Dermatol 2001;45(6):914–8.
68. McGinnis KS, Junkins-Hopkins JM, Crawford G, et al. Low-dose oral bexarotene in combination with low-dose interferon alfa in the treatment of cutaneous T-cell lymphoma: clinical synergism and possible immunologic mechanisms. J Am Acad Dermatol 2004;50(3):375–9.
69. Lee JH, Cheng AL, Lin CW, et al. Multifocal primary cutaneous CD30+ anaplastic large cell lymphoma responsive to thalidomide: the molecular mechanism and the clinical application. Br J Dermatol 2009;160(4):887–9.
70. Duvic M, Talpur R, Wen S, et al. Phase II evaluation of gemcitabine monotherapy for cutaneous T-cell lymphoma. Clin Lymphoma Myeloma 2006;7(1):51–8.
71. Rijlaarsdam JU, Huijgens PC, Beljaards RC, et al. Oral etoposide in the treatment of cutaneous large-cell lymphomas. A preliminary report of four cases. Br J Dermatol 1992;127(5):524–8.
72. Seckin D, Barete S, Euvrard S, et al. Primary cutaneous posttransplant lymphoproliferative disorders in solid organ transplant recipients: a multicenter European case series. Am J Transplant 2013;13(8):2146–53.

Rare Cutaneous T-Cell Lymphomas

Fabiana Damasco, MD, Oleg E. Akilov, MD, PhD*

KEYWORDS

- T-cell lymphomas • CD8 • Gamma/delta T cells • NK cells

KEY POINTS

- Rare lymphoma includes the entities that occur in less than 1% of cases of all lymphomas.
- Although the percentage is low, there are more than eight lymphomas classified as rare lymphomas.
- In this article, the authors discuss only the most common rare lymphomas.

PRIMARY CUTANEOUS γδ T-CELL LYMPHOMA

Primary cutaneous γδ T-cell lymphoma (PCGD-TCL) was recognized as a definitive entity in 2008.[1] γδ T cells are a less frequent population of T cells frequently possessing a cytotoxic phenotype.[2–4] PCGD-TCL carries a more aggressive clinical course and presents a poor prognosis.[5,6]

Clinical Presentation

PCGD-TCL has two distinct clinical presentations: panniculitis-like and disseminated indurated plaques and/or ulceronecrotic nodules frequently on the extremities (**Fig. 1**).[7,8] The later presentation was classified as Ketron-Goodman type of pagetoid reticulosis in the past. Some patients who present with mycosis fungoides like patches may have slightly better overall survival.[2,4,6] Mucosal or other extracutaneous sites may be involved, but lymph nodes, spleen, and bone marrow are usually spared.[3,4] Most patients present with B symptoms.[4] The subcutaneous form of PCGD-TCL in 50% of cases is complicated by a hemophagocytic syndrome (HPS).[3,9]

Morphology

The malignant T cells are medium to large in size. The infiltrate is characterized by three major histologic patterns, which are observed in the samples:[3,5]

Disclosure statement: None declared.
Department of Dermatology, University of Pittsburgh, 3708 Fifth Avenue, 5th Floor, Suite 500.68, Pittsburgh, PA 15213, USA
* Corresponding author.
E-mail address: akilovoe@upmc.edu

Hematol Oncol Clin N Am 33 (2019) 135–148
https://doi.org/10.1016/j.hoc.2018.08.004
hemonc.theclinics.com

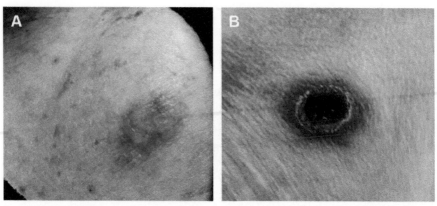

Fig. 1. Primary cutaneous γδ T-cell lymphoma. (*A*) Indurated plaque on the left shoulder. (*B*) Ulcerated nodule on the left breast.

- Epidermotropism from mild to marked, pagetoid reticulosis-like, with extensive necrosis of keratinocytes and ulceration,[7,10,11] the reason why PCGD-TCL was classified as pagetoid reticulosis in the past.
- Involvement of the dermis from mild perivascular to confluent and deep nodular[4] corresponding tumor type of PCGD-TCL.
- Involvement of the subcutaneous tissue with rimming of individual adipocytes corresponding panniculitis-like PCGD-TCL.[4]

Apoptotic cells, areas of angiocentricity, angiodestruction, and tissue necrosis are also common.[4,5,7]

Immunophenotype

The neoplastic T cells are typically positive for TCRγ, CD2, and CD3. Because in many institutions TCRγ stain is not available, the absence of TCRβ positivity (βF1 staining) on malignant cells is considered to be an equivalent of TCRγ phenotype. Some cases have a strong expression of cytotoxic proteins.[3,6,7] The expression of CD4 and CD8 is usually double negative; the maturation markers, such as CD5 and CD7, are frequently lost; and the expression of CD56 is variable.[4] Epstein-Barr virus (EBV) is frequently negative but is positive in isolated cases.[12]

Genetics and Molecular Findings

Although most cases of PCGD-TCL show a monoclonal rearrangement of the TCRγ chain gene,[3,4] TCRγ monoclonality does not equal diagnosis of PCGD-TCL because the presence of rearrangement is not equal to presence of the protein on the surface. TCRγ is frequently positive in conventional αβ cutaneous T-cell lymphoma along with TCRβ. Only TCRδ monoclonality should be used for diagnosis of PCGD-TCL, but this test is not available in most institutions. Thus, TCRγ stain caries higher diagnostic value. Isochromosome 7q is a common genetic abnormality.[13] Küçük and colleagues[14] found that activating mutations of STAT5B N642H is particularly frequent in all forms of γδ-T-cell lymphomas.

Prognosis

The median survival ranges from 15 to 31 months. Patients with subcutaneous fat involvement have a worse prognosis.[4,6,7] The prognosis is gravid even with the limited number of tumors,[4] and no significant differences in survival were found between cases with and without HPS.[7]

Management

Vidulich and colleagues[15] published a study with a successful response and remission of the disease with local radiation followed by weekly infusions of denileukin diftitox. Brentuximab vedotin has been recently reported in cases with relapsed/refractory PCGD-TCL and demonstrated to be effective and well-tolerated.[16,17] Küçük and colleagues[14] found that STAT5B mutations are far more frequent in $\gamma\delta$ T-cell lymphomas, suggesting a pivotal role of STAT5B in the pathogenesis of the disease. This suggest that JAK-STAT pathway inhibition may be a potential therapeutic target.

PRIMARY CUTANEOUS CD4$^+$ SMALL/MEDIUM T-CELL LYMPHOPROLIFERATIVE DISORDER

Primary cutaneous CD4$^+$ small/medium T-cell lymphoproliferative disorder (PCSMTC LPD) remains a provisional entity with benign clinical course accounting for 2% to 3% of all cutaneous T-cell lymphoma.[5]

Clinical Presentation

Most patients with PCSMTCL LPD present with 1- or 2-month history of a solitary nodule (rarely plaque) frequently located on the face and neck (**Fig. 2**A).[18–22] The average age at the time of diagnosis ranges from 50 to 60 years.[18,22] Systemic involvement is absent.[22] The diagnosis of multifocal and disseminated PCSMTCL LPD should be carefully reconsidered in favor of peripheral T-cell lymphoma, not otherwise specified.

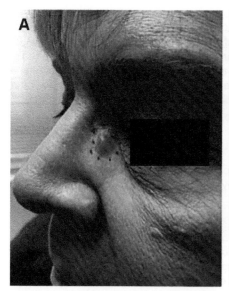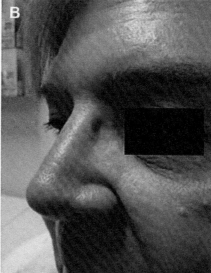

Fig. 2. Primary cutaneous CD4$^+$ small/medium T-cell lymphoproliferative disorder. (*A*) Well-defined bluish nodule on the left upper portion of the nasal sidewall clinically mistaken for basal cell carcinoma. (*B*) Complete resolution after diagnostic punch biopsy 8 months later.

Morphology

The lesions are characterized by dense, nodular, or diffuse dermal infiltrate without significant epidermotropism or folliculotropism.[18–20,23] The small-to medium-sized pleomorphic CD4[+] T cells predominate in the mixed infiltrate of small reactive CD8[+] T cells, B cells, plasma cells, eosinophils, and histiocytes. Multinucleated giant cells can also be found in various numbers.[20,23]

Immunophenotype

The pleomorphic cells express CD3[+] and CD4[+], and almost all cases are CD8[-] and CD30[-]without the expression of cytotoxic markers.[18,20,23] The CD8[+] T cells can constitute up to 5% to 47% of the cells.[24] No surface markers are predictive of an aggressive course, including Ki-67 index, which has a low rate in most patients.[22] Loss of CD5 and CD7 is uncommon. The neoplastic cells are positive for TCRβ.[25] The atypical CD4[+] T cells frequently express follicular T-helper cell markers (programmed death 1, BCL6, and CXCL13),[20,26] suggesting a role of the B-cell activation by follicular T-helper cells in some PCSMTCL LPD cases.[20]

Genetics and Molecular Findings

Most of the cases have monoclonal rearrangement of TCR gene detected.[20,23,26] Specific genetic abnormalities have not been described.

Prognosis

Patients have favorable prognosis and indolent clinical course. Frequent self-resolution after diagnostic punch biopsy was reported (**Fig. 2**B), and durable response to skin-directed medications with rare local recurrence after treatments is common.[18,22,23,26] The 5-year survival rate exceeds 90%.[5,18,19,23]

Management

Some cases may resolve spontaneously after skin biopsy.[20,26] Treatment options for persistent lesions include intralesional steroids, local excision, and low-dose radiotherapy.[18,20,22,26] Resolution following the administration of doxycycline has been reported.[27] Patients usually show a high rate of complete remission, and relapse rates are low after treatment.[21,22]

PRIMARY CUTANEOUS ACRAL CD8[+] T-CELL LYMPHOMA

Primary cutaneous acral CD8[+] T-cell lymphoma (PCA-TCL) is a new indolent provisional entity recognized in the 2016 revision of the World Health Organization classification.[28]

Clinical Presentation

Most patients are men who are 50 and older typically presenting with slow-growing solitary or symmetric bilateral papule or nodule, most commonly located on the ear (**Fig. 3**), but it can also occur on the nose or other acral sites (hands and feet).[3,29–31] Kluk and colleagues[29] reported a case with recurrent and multifocal lesions on acral sites. PCA-TCL has benign course, and systemic involvement has not yet been observed.[29]

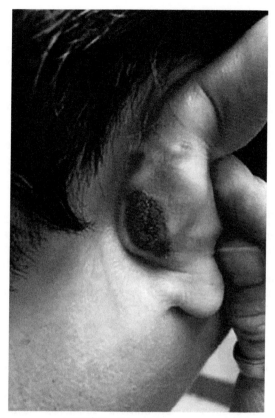

Fig. 3. Primary cutaneous acral CD8[+] T-cell lymphoma.

Morphology

The epidermis is not involved in most cases.[32] Monomorphous, medium-sized CD8[+] cytotoxic T cells form a diffuse dermal infiltrate separated from the epidermis by a Grenz zone.[33] Necrosis, ulceration, and angiocentricity are commonly absent.[30]

Immunophenotyping

The neoplastic cells are positive for CD3, CD8, and TIA-1; and negative for CD4, granzyme B, CD56, and CD30, without the expression of follicular T-cell markers.[21,33] In contrast with the aggressive CD8[+] primary cutaneous T-cell lymphoma, the proliferation index is low in most cases.[3,33,34] Although none of other CD8[+] lymphoma express CD68, in this type of lymphoma, CD68 often shows a positive perinuclear dot-like pattern in the Golgi zone of neoplastic cells and may be used for differential diagnostics.[34]

Molecular Findings

Most cases exhibit a monoclonal TCR rearrangement.[29,30,33]

Prognosis

Prognosis is excellent even in cases of cutaneous relapse.[21,29]

Management

Patients respond well to skin-directed therapy, such as topical and intralesional steroids and radiation.[21,29,30] Excisions are rarely needed. Treatment with interferon, PUVA, and methotrexate has been tested to reduce cutaneous relapses with variable success rates.[29,35]

PRIMARY CUTANEOUS CD8+ AGGRESSIVE EPIDERMOTROPIC CYTOTOXIC T-CELL LYMPHOMA

Most patients with primary cutaneous CD8+ aggressive epidermotropic cytotoxic T-cell lymphoma (PCAE-TCL) are elderly men who often present rapidly progressing disseminated tumors with frequent extracutaneous involvement.[36–38] Prognosis is poor.

Clinical Presentation

PCAE-TCL is characterized by abrupt onset of infiltrated, ulcerated, and hemorrhagic annular infiltrated plaques and nodules disseminated all over the body including the face (**Fig. 4**).[36,37] The lymphoma spreads rapidly metastasizing to the lungs, adrenal glands, testis, and the central nervous system.[36,37,39] Uncommon presentation includes widespread annular erythematous scaling patches[40] and multiple maculopapular plane wartlike eruptions on hands, feet, and face.[41]

Morphology

A considerable epidermotropism frequently presents with a pagetoid spread.[36–38] Focal to confluent keratinocyte necrosis and ulceration are often seen.[38] The various size atypical lymphocytes can infiltrate the dermis deeply, and usually can reach the subcutaneous fat but without adipocyte rimming.[37,38] The findings of angiocentricity, angioinvasion, and destruction of adnexal structures have been reported occasionally.[3,5,37]

Immunophenotype

The malignant T cells usually express CD3+, CD8+, and cytotoxic markers (TIA1, perforin, and granzyme B), negative for CD4, CD45RO, CD2, and CD5.[36,39] CD56 and CD30 showed variable expression.[5,37–40] The Ki-67 proliferation index is usually

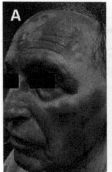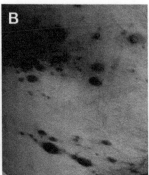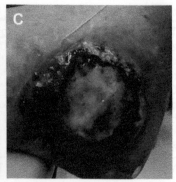

Fig. 4. Primary cutaneous CD8+ aggressive epidermotropic cytotoxic T-cell lymphoma. (*A*) Nodules and indurated plaques with infiltrative pattern on the face. (*B*) Multiple monomorphic tumors on the trunk. (*C*) Ulcerated tumor on the right ankle.

high.[36,39] Guitart and colleagues[38] identified cases with lack of CD8 and cases with αβ/γδ heterodimer expression with similar clinicopathologic presentation, cytotoxicity, and aggressive course as PCAE-TCL. Based on their observation, they suggest that the term "primary cutaneous aggressive epidermotropic cytotoxic T-cell lymphoma" may be better suited.

Genetics and Molecular Findings

The neoplastic T cells show clonal TCR gene rearrangements.[5,37] Specific genetic abnormalities have not been described, but chromosomal instability and haploinsufficiency for TP53 subsequently affecting p14ARF-Mdm2-p53 tumor suppressor protein pathway were observed in PCAE-TCL.[42]

Prognosis

PCAE-TCL has an aggressive clinical course with a median overall survival ranging from 12[36,38] to 32 months.[39] Five-year overall survival rate ranges from 18% to 32%.[37,38]

Management

There are few documented cases that respond to brentuximab vedotin and to pralatrexate showing significant antidisease activity in relapsed/resistant patients with PCAE-TCL.[43] Partial response was reported following oral bexarotene plus total skin electron beam treatment.[44] Interferon is contraindicated because it leads to degranulation of CD8 cytotoxic cells worsening the clinical course. Hematopoietic allogeneic stem cell transplantation seems to be the only therapeutic option associated with some sustained responses and durable remission, and should be included early in the treatment of selected cases of PCAE-TCL.[37,38,43]

EXTRANODAL NK-/T-CELL LYMPHOMA, NASAL TYPE

Extranodal NK-/T-cell lymphoma, nasal type (ENKL) is a rare and aggressive disorder observed in South East Asia and some areas of Central and South America.[3,45] It is a rare lymphoma in the United States and when it happens, it has a higher incidence among Hispanic and Asian/Pacific Islanders.[46,47] ENKL is designated NK/T because most cases have ambiguity in cellular origins with NK-cells and rarely cytotoxic T-cell phenotypes (αβ or γδ T cells).[48] ENKL is nearly always EBV-positive. ENKL affects the lymphoid tissue of the upper respiratory tract (the Waldeyer tonsillar ring), followed by the skin.[1,28] There is a predominance in male patients with a median age at presentation of 52 years; however, rare cases have been reported during childhood.[47,49]

Clinical Presentation

Most patients present with localized disease of the Waldeyer tonsillar ring, resulting in symptoms of nasal obstruction, epistaxis, and/or tumor involving the midface known as "lethal mid-line granuloma" (**Fig. 5**A).[3,28] Although 75% of patients have localized disease at initial presentation, the disease can disseminate rapidly to various sites (skin, gastrointestinal tract, testis, and lymph nodes).[50] The skin is the second most common site of involvement after the nasal cavity/nasopharynx.[45] The most common skin presentation is multiple erythematous to violaceous (usually ulcerated) plaques and tumors on the trunk and extremities (**Fig. 5**B), but it can present as patches, annular plaques, nodules, hydroa vacciniforme-like lesions, chronic ulcers, or subcutaneous infiltrated plaques.[3,45] Lymph nodes and bone marrow may be involved

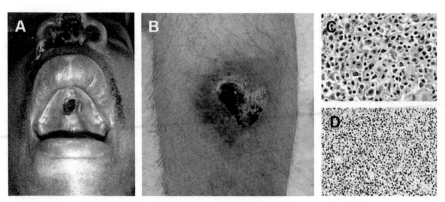

Fig. 5. Extranodal NK-/T-cell lymphoma, nasal type. (*A*) "Lethal mid-line granuloma" involving the nasal cavity and hard palate. (*B*) Ulcerated tumor on the foreleg. (*C*) Large atypical NK/T lymphocytes (hematoxylin-eosin, original magnification ×100). (*D*) EBV-positive malignant lymphocytes (original magnification ×40). ([*A*] *Courtesy of* S. Whitley, MD, PhD, Pittsburgh, PA.)

secondarily. Other extranodal sites (gastrointestinal tract, testis, lung, eye, or soft tissue)[47,49,51] may be involved either primarily or as a direct extension of the primary tumor. Approximately 40% of patients may present with B symptoms.[5,47,49] The disease can be complicated by HPS, which is associated with worse outcomes and a high mortality rate.[52]

Morphology

Histologically, ENKL shows a dense dermal or subcutaneous infiltrate with polymorphic atypical lymphocytes (**Fig. 5**C), along with normal lymphocytes, plasma cells, and occasionally eosinophils and histiocytes.[2,3,5] It is also characteristic, but not essential, an angioinvasive and angiodestructive growth pattern of infiltration often associated with extensive coagulative necrosis of surrounding tissues.[53]

Immunophenotyping

The atypical cells are CD2$^+$, CD56$^+$, and negative for CD4 and for surface CD3, but frequently positive for cytoplasmic CD3.[53] Most of neoplastic cells also contain the cytotoxic granules-associated proteins.[3,53] Although CD56 is typically expressed, in cases of negative CD56, both the expression of cytotoxic molecules and a positive EBV are required for diagnosis of ENKL.[1] Uncommon cases may express CD4, CD8, and/or CD7.[48] Monoclonal EBV-DNA genomes and detectable EBV-encoded small nuclear RNAs by in situ hybridization technique (**Fig. 5**D) are virtually present in all cases.[3,51]

Genetic and Molecular Findings

Clonal rearrangement of the TCR genes is seen in T-cell-derived ENKTL cases. Molecular analyses have found frequent inactivation of tumor suppressor genes, such as PRDM1, TP53, TP73, DDX3X, and PTPN6 (SHP1). BCL2L11 (BIM) is often methylated and activating mutations of STAT3 and, less frequently, STAT5B have been described.[3,14]

Prognosis

ENKL has an aggressive clinical course with a poor prognosis. Without treatment, most patients die within a few months of diagnosis (median survival, 15 months).[5] Some studies have reported that high levels of EBV in the plasma or bone marrow apparently can predict a worse outcome.[51] Additional poor prognosis factors are extranasal presentation, advanced stage, performance status, and number of extra-nodal involved sites.[54,55]

Management

For patients with localized disease, high-dose radiotherapy should be considered as the first choice of treatment. Multiagent chemotherapy does not provide prolonged remission, does not improve overall survival significantly, and is associated with high mortality rate. Allogeneic Hematopoietic Cell Transplantation is recommended as early as possible.[2] The efficacy of anti–programmed death 1 inhibitors has been reported in the therapy for ENKL.[56]

SUBCUTANEOUS PANNICULITIS-LIKE T-CELL LYMPHOMA

According to the World Health Organization/European Organisation for Research and Treatment of Cancer classification, subcutaneous panniculitis-like T-cell lymphoma (SPTCL) is restricted to cases of $\alpha\beta$ T lymphocytes only.[5,28,57] Differentiation from lupus panniculitis may present significant difficulties, and some cases exhibit overlap especially in patients with known history of autoimmune disease.[7,58]

Clinical Presentation

Most cases arise in young women, with median age at presentation of 36 years.[7] SPTCL presents multiple, subcutaneous, inflammatory nodules or indurated plaques usually on the lower extremities, but SPTCL can affect the trunk (**Fig. 6**A) and upper

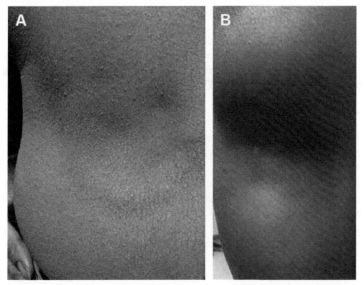

Fig. 6. Subcutaneous panniculitis-like T-cell lymphoma. (*A*) Subcutaneous indurated plaque on the trunk. (*B*) Subcutaneous indurated plaque on the left shoulder.

extremities (**Fig. 6**B), and less commonly the face.[2,7] Ulceration is uncommon and disseminated disease is extremely rare.[7] Nodal and visceral involvement is rare. A spontaneous waxing-and-waning course is common.[45] About 20% of patients may develop HPS, which worsens their overall good prognosis.[7,59]

Morphology

Pleomorphic small- to medium-sized T cells are predominant and an often exclusive component of the cellular infiltrate in the subcutaneous fat lobules, generally sparing the overlying epidermis, dermis, and adnexal structures.[7] Extensive areas with fat necrosis, cytophagocytosis, and karyorrhexis may be present.[60] A characteristic, but not exclusive, histopathologic feature is the rimming of the individual fat cells by neoplastic lymphocytes.[61]

Immunophenotyping

SPTCL typically express CD2, CD3, and TCRαβ phenotype and are negative for CD4 and CD56.[62] In most cases (75%),[7] neoplastic cells are positive for CD8 often with loss of CD2, CD5, and CD7.[7] There is an intense, diffuse positivity for the cytotoxic granular proteins (TIA-1, perforin, and granzyme B) in almost all cases.[2]

Genetics and Molecular Findings

Clonal rearrangement of the TCRγ and β genes is frequently detected.[7] No specific cytogenetic abnormalities have been described.[1,2]

Prognosis

Most patients present an indolent clinical course with a 5-year survival rate of more than 80%.[7] Patients with HPS have a significantly worse prognosis with a 5-year overall survival rate of 46%.[7] Other factors reported in association with unfavorable prognosis are low white blood cell count or elevated lactate dehydrogenase.[59]

Management

Patients with indolent forms usually respond to systemic corticosteroids, oral methotrexate, or oral bexarotene.[7,63,64] Other systemic agents found to be beneficial are histone deacetylase inhibitors and denileukin diftitox.[65] In cases of solitary or localized disease, radiotherapy is recommended alone or in combination with other systemic agents.[2,45] Because there is significant overlap with lupus panniculitis, previous studies have suggested that cyclosporine A might have some efficacy for relapsed or initial SPTCL.[66,67]

REFERENCES

1. Swerdlow SH, Campo E, Harris NL, et al. WHO Classification of Tumours of Haematopoietic and Lymphoid Tissues. 4th Edition. Lyon (France): International Agency for Research on Cancer; 2008.
2. Gallardo F, Pujol RM. Subcutaneous panniculitic-like T-cell lymphoma and other primary cutaneous lymphomas with prominent subcutaneous tissue involvement. Dermatol Clin 2008;26(4):529–40.
3. Rubio-Gonzalez B, Zain J, Rosen ST, et al. Clinical manifestations and pathogenesis of cutaneous lymphomas: current status and future directions. Br J Haematol 2017;176(1):16–36.
4. Guitart J, Weisenburger DD, Subtil A, et al. Cutaneous γδ T-cell lymphomas: a spectrum of presentations with overlap with other cytotoxic lymphomas. Am J Surg Pathol 2012;36(11):1656–65.

5. Willemze R, Jaffe ES, Burg G, et al. WHO-EORTC classification for cutaneous lymphomas. Blood 2005;105(10):3768–85.
6. Toro JR, Liewehr DJ, Pabby N, et al. Gamma-delta T-cell phenotype is associated with significantly decreased survival in cutaneous T-cell lymphoma. Blood 2003; 101(9):3407–12.
7. Willemze R, Jansen PM, Cerroni L, et al. Subcutaneous panniculitis-like T-cell lymphoma: definition, classification, and prognostic factors: an EORTC Cutaneous Lymphoma Group Study of 83 cases. Blood 2008;111(2):838–45.
8. Endly DC, Weenig RH, Peters MS, et al. Indolent course of cutaneous gamma-delta T-cell lymphoma. J Cutan Pathol 2013;40(10):896–902.
9. Mehta-Shah N, Horwitz S. Uncommon variants of T-cell lymphomas. Hematol Oncol Clin North Am 2017;31(2):285–95.
10. Toro JR, Beaty M, Sorbara L, et al. Gamma delta T-cell lymphoma of the skin: a clinical, microscopic, and molecular study. Arch Dermatol 2000;136(8):1024–32.
11. Berti E, Cerri A, Cavicchini S, et al. Primary cutaneous gamma/delta T-cell lymphoma presenting as disseminated pagetoid reticulosis. J Invest Dermatol 1991;96(5):718–23.
12. Yu W-W, Hsieh P-P, Chuang S-S. Cutaneous EBV-positive $\gamma\delta$ T-cell lymphoma vs. extranodal NK/T-cell lymphoma: a case report and literature review. J Cutan Pathol 2013;40(3):310–6.
13. Kempf W, Kazakov DV, Kerl K. Cutaneous lymphomas: an update. Part 1: T-cell and natural killer/t-cell lymphomas and related conditions. Am J Dermatopathol 2014;36(2):105–23.
14. Küçük C, Jiang B, Hu X, et al. Activating mutations of STAT5B and STAT3 in lymphomas derived from $\gamma\delta$-T or NK cells. Nat Commun 2015;6:6025.
15. Vidulich K, Jones D, Duvic M. Cutaneous γ/δ T-cell lymphoma treated with radiation and denileukin diftitox. Clin Lymphoma Myeloma 2008;8(1):55–8.
16. Talpur R, Chockalingam R, Wang C, et al. A single-center experience with brentuximab vedotin in gamma delta T-cell lymphoma. Clin Lymphoma Myeloma Leuk 2016;16(2):e15–9.
17. Rubio-Gonzalez B, Zain J, Garcia L, et al. Cutaneous gamma-delta T-cell lymphoma successfully treated with brentuximab vedotin. JAMA Dermatol 2016; 152(12):1388–90.
18. Grogg KL, Jung S, Erickson LA, et al. Primary cutaneous CD4-positive small/medium-sized pleomorphic T-cell lymphoma: a clonal T-cell lymphoproliferative disorder with indolent behavior. Mod Pathol 2008;21(6):708–15.
19. Garcia-Herrera A, Colomo L, Camós M, et al. Primary cutaneous small/medium CD4+ T-cell lymphomas: a heterogeneous group of tumors with different clinicopathologic features and outcome. J Clin Oncol 2008;26(20):3364–71.
20. Rodríguez Pinilla SM, Roncador G, Rodríguez-Peralto JL, et al. Primary cutaneous CD4+ small/medium-sized pleomorphic T-cell lymphoma expresses follicular T-cell markers. Am J Surg Pathol 2009;33(1):81–90.
21. Virmani P, Jawed S, Myskowski PL, et al. Long-term follow-up and management of small and medium-sized CD4+ T cell lymphoma and CD8+ lymphoid proliferations of acral sites: a multicenter experience. Int J Dermatol 2016;55(11): 1248–54.
22. James E, Sokhn JG, Gibson JF, et al. CD4 + primary cutaneous small/medium-sized pleomorphic T-cell lymphoma: a retrospective case series and review of literature. Leuk Lymphoma 2015;56(4):951–7.
23. Beltraminelli H, Leinweber B, Kerl H, et al. Primary cutaneous CD4+ small-/medium-sized pleomorphic T-cell lymphoma: a cutaneous nodular proliferation of

pleomorphic T lymphocytes of undetermined significance? A study of 136 cases. Am J Dermatopathol 2009;31(4):317–22.

24. Lan TTH, Brown NA, Hristov AC. Controversies and considerations in the diagnosis of primary cutaneous CD4$^+$ small/medium T-cell lymphoma. Arch Pathol Lab Med 2014;138(10):1307–18.

25. Gru AA, Wick MR, Eid M. Primary cutaneous CD4+ small/medium T-cell lymphoproliferative disorder-clinical and histopathologic features, differential diagnosis, and treatment. Semin Cutan Med Surg 2018;37(1):39–48.

26. Cetinözman F, Jansen PM, Willemze R. Expression of programmed death-1 in primary cutaneous CD4-positive small/medium-sized pleomorphic T-cell lymphoma, cutaneous pseudo-T-cell lymphoma, and other types of cutaneous T-cell lymphoma. Am J Surg Pathol 2012;36(1):109–16.

27. Toberer F, Hartschuh W, Hadaschik E. Primary cutaneous CD4+ small- to medium-sized pleomorphic T-cell lymphoma: temporary remission by oral doxycycline. JAMA Dermatol 2013;149(8):956–9.

28. Swerdlow SH, Campo E, Pileri SA, et al. The 2016 revision of the World Health Organization classification of lymphoid neoplasms. Blood 2016;127(20):2375–90.

29. Kluk J, Kai A, Koch D, et al. Indolent CD8-positive lymphoid proliferation of acral sites: three further cases of a rare entity and an update on a unique patient. J Cutan Pathol 2016;43(2):125–36.

30. Greenblatt D, Ally M, Child F, et al. Indolent CD8(+) lymphoid proliferation of acral sites: a clinicopathologic study of six patients with some atypical features. J Cutan Pathol 2013;40(2):248–58.

31. Wobser M, Petrella T, Kneitz H, et al. Extrafacial indolent CD8-positive cutaneous lymphoid proliferation with unusual symmetrical presentation involving both feet. J Cutan Pathol 2013;40(11):955–61.

32. Hathuc VM, Hristov AC, Smith LB. Primary cutaneous acral CD8+ T-cell lymphoma. Arch Pathol Lab Med 2017;141(11):1469–75.

33. Petrella T, Maubec E, Cornillet-Lefebvre P, et al. Indolent CD8-positive lymphoid proliferation of the ear: a distinct primary cutaneous T-cell lymphoma? Am J Surg Pathol 2007;31(12):1887–92.

34. Wobser M, Roth S, Reinartz T, et al. CD68 expression is a discriminative feature of indolent cutaneous CD8-positive lymphoid proliferation and distinguishes this lymphoma subtype from other CD8-positive cutaneous lymphomas. Br J Dermatol 2015;172(6):1573–80.

35. Kempf W, Kazakov DV, Cozzio A, et al. Primary cutaneous CD8(+) small- to medium-sized lymphoproliferative disorder in extrafacial sites: clinicopathologic features and concept on their classification. Am J Dermatopathol 2013;35(2):159–66.

36. Robson A, Assaf C, Bagot M, et al. Aggressive epidermotropic cutaneous CD8+ lymphoma: a cutaneous lymphoma with distinct clinical and pathological features. Report of an EORTC Cutaneous Lymphoma Task Force Workshop. Histopathology 2015;67(4):425–41.

37. Nofal A, Abdel-Mawla MY, Assaf M, et al. Primary cutaneous aggressive epidermotropic CD8+ T-cell lymphoma: proposed diagnostic criteria and therapeutic evaluation. J Am Acad Dermatol 2012;67(4):748–59.

38. Guitart J, Martinez-Escala ME, Subtil A, et al. Primary cutaneous aggressive epidermotropic cytotoxic T-cell lymphomas: reappraisal of a provisional entity in the 2016 WHO classification of cutaneous lymphomas. Mod Pathol 2017;30(5):761–72.

39. Berti E, Tomasini D, Vermeer MH, et al. Primary cutaneous CD8-positive epidermotropic cytotoxic T cell lymphomas. A distinct clinicopathological entity with an aggressive clinical behavior. Am J Pathol 1999;155(2):483–92.
40. Yoshizawa N, Yagi H, Horibe T, et al. Primary cutaneous aggressive epidermotropic CD8+ T-cell lymphoma with a CD15(+)CD30(-) phenotype. Eur J Dermatol 2007;17(5):441–2.
41. Kim SK, Kim YC, Kang HY. Primary cutaneous aggressive epidermotropic CD8(+) cytotoxic T-cell lymphoma with atypical presentation. J Dermatol 2006; 33(9):632–4.
42. Kato K, Oh Y, Takita J, et al. Molecular genetic and cytogenetic analysis of a primary cutaneous CD8-positive aggressive epidermotropic cytotoxic T-cell lymphoma. Int J Hematol 2016;103(2):196–201.
43. Cyrenne BM, Gibson JF, Subtil A, et al. Transplantation in the treatment of primary cutaneous aggressive epidermotropic cytotoxic CD8-positive T-cell lymphoma. Clin Lymphoma Myeloma Leuk 2018;18(1):e85–93.
44. Gormley RH, Hess SD, Anand D, et al. Primary cutaneous aggressive epidermotropic CD8+ T-cell lymphoma. J Am Acad Dermatol 2010;62(2):300–7.
45. Willemze R, Hodak E, Zinzani PL, et al, ESMO Guidelines Working Group. Primary cutaneous lymphomas: ESMO Clinical Practice Guidelines for diagnosis, treatment and follow-up. Ann Oncol 2013;24(Suppl 6):vi149–54.
46. Adams SV, Newcomb PA, Shustov AR. Racial patterns of peripheral T-cell lymphoma incidence and survival in the United States. J Clin Oncol 2016;34(9): 963–71.
47. Au W, Weisenburger DD, Intragumtornchai T, et al. Clinical differences between nasal and extranasal natural killer/T-cell lymphoma: a study of 136 cases from the International Peripheral T-Cell Lymphoma Project. Blood 2009;113(17): 3931–7.
48. Pongpruttipan T, Sukpanichnant S, Assanasen T, et al. Extranodal NK/T-cell lymphoma, nasal type, includes cases of natural killer cell and αβ, γδ, and αβ/γδ T-cell origin: a comprehensive clinicopathologic and phenotypic study. Am J Surg Pathol 2012;36(4):481–99.
49. Li Y-X, Liu Q-F, Fang H, et al. Variable clinical presentations of nasal and Waldeyer ring natural killer/T-cell lymphoma. Clin Cancer Res 2009;15(8):2905–12.
50. Makita S, Tobinai K. Clinical features and current optimal management of natural killer/T-cell lymphoma. Hematol Oncol Clin North Am 2017;31(2):239–53.
51. Lei KIK, Chan LYS, Chan W-Y, et al. Diagnostic and prognostic implications of circulating cell-free Epstein-Barr virus DNA in natural killer/T-cell lymphoma. Clin Cancer Res 2002;8(1):29–34.
52. Han A-R, Lee HR, Park B-B, et al. Lymphoma-associated hemophagocytic syndrome: clinical features and treatment outcome. Ann Hematol 2007;86(7):493–8.
53. Jaffe ES, Chan JK, Su IJ, et al. Report of the workshop on nasal and related extranodal angiocentric T/natural killer cell lymphomas. Definitions, differential diagnosis, and epidemiology. Am J Surg Pathol 1996;20(1):103–11.
54. Suzuki R, Suzumiya J, Yamaguchi M, et al. Prognostic factors for mature natural killer (NK) cell neoplasms: aggressive NK cell leukemia and extranodal NK cell lymphoma, nasal type. Ann Oncol 2010;21(5):1032–40.
55. Bekkenk MW, Jansen PM, Meijer CJLM, et al. CD56+ hematological neoplasms presenting in the skin: a retrospective analysis of 23 new cases and 130 cases from the literature. Ann Oncol 2004;15(7):1097–108.

56. Kwong Y-L, Chan TSY, Tan D, et al. PD1 blockade with pembrolizumab is highly effective in relapsed or refractory NK/T-cell lymphoma failing l-asparaginase. Blood 2017;129(17):2437–42.
57. Massone C, Lozzi GP, Egberts F, et al. The protean spectrum of non-Hodgkin lymphomas with prominent involvement of subcutaneous fat. J Cutan Pathol 2006; 33(6):418–25.
58. Hahtola S, Burghart E, Jeskanen L, et al. Clinicopathological characterization and genomic aberrations in subcutaneous panniculitis-like T-cell lymphoma. J Invest Dermatol 2008;128(9):2304–9.
59. Go RS, Wester SM. Immunophenotypic and molecular features, clinical outcomes, treatments, and prognostic factors associated with subcutaneous panniculitis-like T-cell lymphoma: a systematic analysis of 156 patients reported in the literature. Cancer 2004;101(6):1404–13.
60. Jaffe ES, Nicolae A, Pittaluga S. Peripheral T-cell and NK-cell lymphomas in the WHO classification: pearls and pitfalls. Mod Pathol 2013;26(Suppl 1):S71–87.
61. Lozzi GP, Massone C, Citarella L, et al. Rimming of adipocytes by neoplastic lymphocytes: a histopathologic feature not restricted to subcutaneous T-cell lymphoma. Am J Dermatopathol 2006;28(1):9–12.
62. Weenig RH, Ng CS, Perniciaro C. Subcutaneous panniculitis-like T-cell lymphoma: an elusive case presenting as lipomembranous panniculitis and a review of 72 cases in the literature. Am J Dermatopathol 2001;23(3):206–15.
63. Briki H, Bouaziz JD, Molinier-Frenkel V, et al. Subcutaneous panniculitis-like T-cell lymphoma αβ: complete sustained remission with corticosteroids and methotrexate. Br J Dermatol 2010;163(5):1136–8.
64. Mehta N, Wayne AS, Kim YH, et al. Bexarotene is active against subcutaneous panniculitis-like T-cell lymphoma in adult and pediatric populations. Clin Lymphoma Myeloma Leuk 2012;12(1):20–5.
65. Hathaway T, Subtil A, Kuo P, et al. Efficacy of denileukin diftitox in subcutaneous panniculitis-like T-cell lymphoma. Clin Lymphoma Myeloma 2007;7(8):541–5.
66. Lee WS, Hwang J-H, Kim MJ, et al. Cyclosporine a as a primary treatment for panniculitis-like T cell lymphoma: a case with a long-term remission. Cancer Res Treat 2014;46(3):312–6.
67. Jung HR, Yun SY, Choi JH, et al. Cyclosporine in relapsed subcutaneous panniculitis-like T-cell lymphoma after autologous hematopoietic stem cell transplantation. Cancer Res Treat 2011;43(4):255–9.

Cutaneous B-Cell Lymphoma

Amrita Goyal, MD[a], Robert E. LeBlanc, MD[b], Joi B. Carter, MD[c],*

KEYWORDS

- Primary cutaneous B-cell lymphoma • Primary cutaneous marginal zone lymphoma
- Primary cutaneous follicle center lymphoma
- Primary cutaneous diffuse large B-cell lymphoma
- Intravascular large B-cell lymphoma

KEY POINTS

- There are 3 types of primary cutaneous B-cell lymphoma: primary cutaneous marginal zone lymphoma (pcMZL), primary cutaneous follicle center lymphoma (pcFCL), and primary cutaneous diffuse large B-cell lymphoma (pcDLBCL), leg-type.
- pcMZL and pcFCL are generally indolent and have minimal risk of extracutaneous spread, whereas pcDLBCL may be more aggressive.
- Skin biopsy is critical to the diagnosis of cutaneous B-cell lymphomas.

PRIMARY CUTANEOUS B-CELL LYMPHOMAS

Primary cutaneous B-cell lymphomas (pcBCLs) are non-Hodgkin B-cell lymphomas originating in the skin without evidence of extracutaneous disease at presentation.[1] In the United States, pcBCLs make up approximately 25% of all primary cutaneous lymphomas, the remainder predominantly T-cell lymphomas. In general, these lymphomas are more common in men than women and are more common with increasing age.[2] Understanding of the pcBCLs has substantially evolved over time with advancements in molecular studies and immunobiology, and classification was revolutionized by the consensus statement between the World Health Organization (WHO) and European Organisation for the Research and Treatment of Cancer in 2005. The classification presented in this article is based on the updated 2016 WHO classification.[3,4] This consensus classification includes 3 main types of pcBCL: primary cutaneous marginal zone lymphoma (pcMZL), primary cutaneous follicle center lymphoma (pcFCL), and primary cutaneous diffuse large B-cell lymphoma (pcDLBCL), leg-type. Intravascular

Conflicts of Interest: The authors declare no conflicts of interest.
[a] Department of Dermatology, University of Minnesota, 420 Delaware Street Southeast, Minneapolis, MN 55401, USA; [b] Department of Pathology and Laboratory Medicine, Dartmouth Hitchcock Medical Center, One Medical Center Drive, Lebanon, NH 03756, USA; [c] Section of Dermatology, Dartmouth Hitchcock Medical Center, One Medical Center Drive, Lebanon, NH 03756, USA
* Corresponding author.
E-mail address: Joi.B.Carter@hitchcock.org

Hematol Oncol Clin N Am 33 (2019) 149–161
https://doi.org/10.1016/j.hoc.2018.08.006
hemonc.theclinics.com
0889-8588/19/© 2018 Elsevier Inc. All rights reserved.

large B-cell lymphoma (IVLBCL) is also included with the B-cell lymphomas because it is most commonly diagnosed on skin biopsy, although it is not primarily cutaneous. The indolent lymphomas include pcMZL and pcFCL, whereas pcDLBCL and IVLBCL are intermediate to aggressive.

Primary Cutaneous Marginal Zone B-Cell Lymphoma

pcMZL appears in the revised WHO classification of lymphomas under the category of extranodal marginal zone lymphoma of mucosa-associated lymphoid tissue (MALT). It is the second most common pcBCL.[4] The skin is the second most common site for MALT-type lymphomas after the gastrointestinal tract.[5] This indolent non-Hodgkin lymphoma accounts for approximately 25% of patients with pcBCL.[2] The median age for patients with pcMZL lymphoma is 50 years to 53 years, with a range of 6 years to 93 years old.[6–9] It occurs more than twice as often in men than in women.[6–8]

Clinical presentation

Classically, pcMZL presents as solitary or clustered deep-seated, red to violaceous, indurated plaques, nodules, or tumors (**Fig. 1**). These lesions may have surrounding annular or diffuse erythema.[5,6,10] The lesions of pcMZL are most commonly located on the trunk (46%–60%), upper extremities (17%), and face and scalp (13%).[6,7,11] A majority of patients present with either a single lesion (28%–59%) or multifocal regional lesions (24%–72%) and are otherwise asymptomatic. Only 0% to 17% of patients present with disseminated cutaneous lesions.

Histopathology

There are 2 distinct subsets of pcMZL[12,13] (**Fig. 2**). Both are characterized by nodular and diffuse, bottom-heavy dermal lymphoid infiltrates that extend to the subcutis and usually spare the epidermis. The subset without heavy chain class switching resembles extracutaneous MALT lymphomas with sheets of neoplastic B cells. The class switched subset exhibits a polymorphous infiltrate similar to reactive lymphoid hyperplasias. Both pcMZL subtypes may be accompanied by mature germinal center follicles or germinal center residua colonized by lymphoma cells. Cytomorphologically, the neoplastic B cells are small and appear monocytoid, cleaved, or round. Rarely, pcMZL can undergo transformation to an aggressive phenotype characterized by

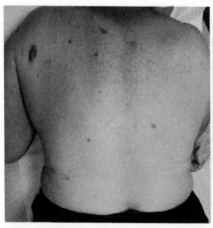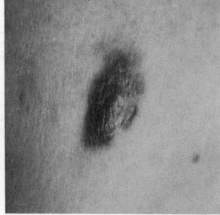

Fig. 1. pcMZL. Scattered reddish-pink smooth papules and plaque of pcMZL on the back (*Left*). Infiltrated plaque of pcMZL (*Right*).

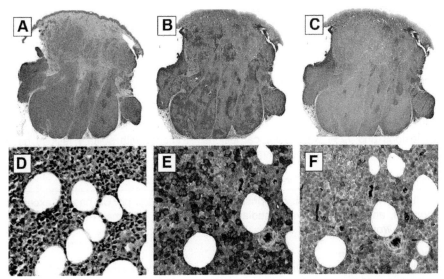

Fig. 2. pcMZL with plasmacytic differentiation. (*A*) A dense, nodular, bottom-heavy lymphoid infiltrate in the reticular dermis and subcutis (hematoxylin-eosin [H&E], ×10). (*B*) Kappa light chain expression (×10) and (*C*) lambda (×10). (*D*) Lymphoid infiltrate with extensive plasmacytic differentiation (H&E, ×200) showing a preponderance of (*E*) kappa expression (×200) and (*F*) rare lambda expression (×200).

blastic cytomorphology,[14] although blastoid features present in pcMZL at disease onset do not necessarily portend aggressive behavior.[15] Both pcMZL subtypes can show variable plasmacytic differentiation, ranging from scattered plasma cells to exclusive plasmacytoid differentiation (formerly called immunocytoma). Plasma cell atypia, including binucleated forms and Dutcher bodies, are common in most cases of pcMZL that show plasmacytic differentiation. Demonstration of a light chain restriction by immunohistochemistry or in situ hybridization is the most sensitive method for establishing clonality in pcMZL.[8,16]

Immunohistochemistry
The immunophenotype (BCL2$^+$, BCL6$^-$, CD10$^-$) of pcMZL helps distinguish pcMZL from pcFCL; however, it cannot distinguish pcMZL from lymphoid hyperplasia or indolent T-cell–rich lymphoid processes. Cases of extensive plasma cell differentiation can show loss of CD20 but express other mature B-cell markers, including CD79a and CD19.[17] CD5 is generally negative, except for rare cases of transformed blastic pcMZL, and otherwise helps distinguish pcMZL from chronic lymphocytic leukemia/small cell lymphoma and mantle cell lymphoma. In contrast with diffuse large B-cell lymphoma (DLBCL), pcMZL comprises small cells and Ki-67 is generally low. The t(14;18) translocation between *IGH* and *MALT1* common to MALT lymphomas is present in only a minority of pcMZLs.[18]

Etiology
Although some studies in European populations suggest an association between pcMZL and *Borrelia burgdorferi*, analogous to the role of *Helicobacter pylori* in gastric MALT lymphoma, this has not been borne out in North American or Asian studies.[7] A

recent study demonstrated an increased incidence of gastrointestinal disorders and autoimmunity in patients with pcMZL compared with a control group.[19]

Prognosis

pcMZL rarely exhibits extracutaneous spread.[6,20] Nodal dissemination and large cell transformation have been reported[21] but disease is skin-limited in a vast majority of patients.[6,7,22] There is a 5-year overall survival of approximately 97%.[22] Complete response to therapy occurs in 93% of patients with solitary lesions and 75% with multifocal disease.[6] Relapses are common within 5 years occurring in 39% with solitary lesions and 77% with multifocal lesions.[6] Patients with solitary lesions have improved survival over those with multifocal disease.[7,22]

Primary Cutaneous Follicle Center Lymphoma

pcFCL is an indolent pcBCL comprising 60% of pcBCLs. pcFCL has an excellent prognosis, and patients have a median age of 50; it is 1.5 times more common in men than women.[23]

Clinical presentation

pcFCL is characterized by slow-growing, 2 cm to 5 cm, firm, smooth, erythematous-to-violaceous plaques, nodules, or tumors. These are rarely ulcerated and often have telangiectasias.[23–25] The tumors primarily occur on the head and neck (61%), upper extremities (23%), and trunk (16%)[23,24] (**Fig. 3**). Most patients have localized or regional disease, with 20% present with unilesional disease and 80% with multiple lesions.[23–25] Although untreated lesions continue to grow, extracutaneous spread is rare (<10%).[23]

Three patterns of cutaneous involvement have been noted: a solitary nodule or plaque on the scalp or trunk[23]; infiltrated papules and plaques on the back, termed Crosti lymphoma[26,27]; and rarely miliary agminated papules.[26,28] Despite morphologic

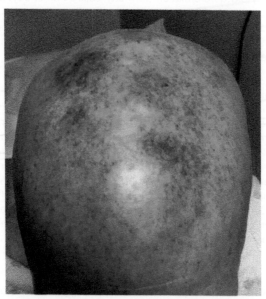

Fig. 3. pcFCL. Scattered pinkish-violet, telangiectatic, smooth, ill-defined patches and thin plaques on the scalp.

differences, these variants of pcFCL all have an excellent prognosis and further sub-division is not necessary.[26]

Histopathology

pcFCL is characterized by irregular, overlapping nodules recapitulating follicles or diffuse sheets of medium-sized B cells with a germinal center phenotype (**Fig. 4**). Tumors involve the dermis and subcutis.[4] Classically, follicles show loss of polarization with an underdeveloped or absent mantle zone, an absence of tingible body macrophages, extension of neoplastic cells beyond follicular dendritic cell networks, and low proliferation. The neoplastic cells resemble cleaved centrocytes with a variable number of centroblasts. In contrast with nodal follicular lymphomas, pcFCL is not assigned a histologic grade based on architecture and cytomorphology.[25] Sheets of centroblasts and immunoblasts, significant cytologic atypia, and increased mitotic activity with single cell necrosis should raise consideration for a more aggressive phenotype. Rarely, pcFCL demonstrates bizarre Reed-Sternberg–like cells[29] or spindle cell appearance that does not affect prognosis.[30–32]

Immunohistochemistry

Immunohistochemical findings are variable: all cases definitionally express germinal center markers, most often BCL6 with varied and heterogeneous coexpression of CD10, STMN1, LMO2, HGAL, and AID.[33] Germinal center differentiation distinguishes pcFCL from pcMZL, and CD21 highlights the underlying follicular dendritic cell networks. BCL2 may be negative or positive in pcFCL and cannot reliably distinguish pcFCL from nodal follicular lymphomas; furthermore, *BCL2* rearrangements can be identified in both of these lymphomas, albeit occurrence is lower in pcFCL.[34] In contrast with pcDLBCL, Ki-67 expression is low in pcFCL and less than 30% of the

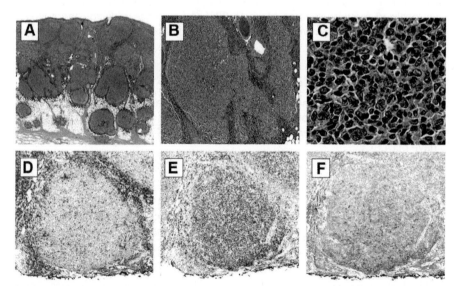

Fig. 4. pcFCL. (*A*) Overlapping, variably sized and shaped nodules reminiscent of reactive germinal center follicles in the reticular dermis and subcutis (H&E, ×10). (*B*) The abnormal follicles lack polarity and mantle zones (H&E, ×40). (*C*) Enlarged, neoplastic centrocytes with cleaved nuclei and scattered centroblasts with conspicuous nucleoli (H&E, ×400). (*D*) Neoplastic follicles are BCL2 negative (×40), (*E*) BCL6 positive (×40), and (*F*) faintly CD10 positive (×40).

B cells expresses MUM1, FOX-P1, IgM, and p63.[35,36] The neoplastic follicles of pcFCL can resemble reactive, hyperplastic germinal center follicles; however, the latter show high Ki-67 expression. Kappa and lambda immunohistochemistry is generally unhelpful in pcFCL; however, IgH gene rearrangement studies can confirm clonality when necessary.

Prognosis

Prognosis for pcFCL is excellent, with a 95% disease-specific 5-year survival rate, with some estimates higher.[23] With treatment, 99% of patients enter complete remission and although 30% experience recurrence, only 10% progress to extracutaneous involvement and cutaneous relapse does not indicate disease progression.[25] Prognosis does not correlate with histologic growth pattern or multifocal disease.[23,25] Location of pcFCL on the leg versus other body sites has been associated with worse overall 5-year survival (22% vs 92%, respectively).[25] Only rare examples of pcFCL transforming to an aggressive DLBCL have been reported.[37]

Staging and Treatment of Indolent Cutaneous B-Cell Lymphoma

Given the clinical, histologic, and immunohistochemical overlap between nodal and cutaneous lymphomas, screening for systemic disease in patients with a new cutaneous lymphoma is recommended. NCCN guidelines for work-up of pcMZL and pcFCL include physical examination, complete blood cell count (CBC) with differential, comprehensive metabolic panel, lactate dehydrogenase (LDH), and CT of the chest/abdomen/pelvis with contrast.[38]

No standardized treatment protocol exists for indolent pcBCLs. Treatments include intralesional steroids, radiotherapy, and excision. Radiation therapy has excellent clearance rates of up to 90%,[39] whereas surgical excision has been reported to have localized recurrence rates of up to 33%.[24] Low-dose radiation therapy was recently reported as effective as standard-dose radiation therapy for the treatment of indolent pcBCL.[39]

Primary Cutaneous Diffuse Large B-Cell Lymphoma, Leg-Type

pcDLBCL, leg type, comprises 10% to 20% of pcBCL and 2.6% of cutaneous lymphomas.[2,40,41] Median age of onset is in the 70s. Asians and Pacific Islanders are at increased risk of pcDLBCL, and women are 2 times to 4 times more likely than men to have pcDLBCL.

Clinical presentation

pcDLBCL, leg type, commonly presents as 2-cm to 5-cm erythematous to violaceous tumors or nodules on the leg, with 10% to 15% on nonleg locations[24,40,42] (**Fig. 5**). Patients generally have a single lesion or grouping of lesions at diagnosis. Patients with leg involvement have higher rates of extracutaneous spread than those with lesions at other sites (33% vs 18%).[43]

Histopathology

pcDLBCL is composed of sheets of large and often monomorphous lymphoid cells with an activated B-cell phenotype (**Fig. 6**). Infiltrates fill the dermis, can involve the subcutis, and occasionally extends to an ulcerated epidermis. The absence of small lymphocytes and granulocytes favors a diagnosis of pcDLBCL over a case of pcFCL with many centroblasts. The cells comprising pcDLBCL show an immunoblastic, centroblastic, or mixed appearance with frequent mitoses.

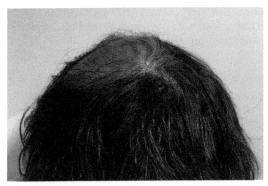

Fig. 5. DLBCL, leg type. Isolated 5-cm × 8-cm reddish-pink indurated tumor with scattered telangiectasia on the vertex scalp.

Immunohistochemistry

In contrast with low-grade B-cell lymphomas, a majority of pcDLBCL cells express Ki-67 and most express activated B-cell markers BCL2 and MUM1. FOX-P1, IgM, and p63-positivity in greater than 30% of the lymphoid infiltrate could also help distinguish pcDLBCL from pcFCL when necessary.[35,36] BCL6 expression is variable between cases of pcDLBCL and rare cases of pcDLBCL lack BCL2 expression. These cases show similar behavior to pcDLBCL with a conventional immunophenotype.[44] CD21-positive follicular dendritic cell networks are not present in pcDLBCL. Epstein-Barr encoding region (EBER) in situ hybridization is negative in pcDLBCL and should be performed to exclude an Epstein-Barr virus–associated DLBCL. A majority of cases of pcDLBCL contain a 9p21.3 deletion, including the *CDKN2A* and *CDKN2B* loci.[45]

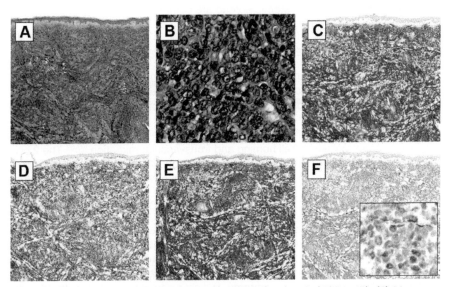

Fig. 6. DLBCL, leg type. (*A*) Dense sheets of cells in the dermis (H&E, ×10). (*B*) Monomorphous infiltrate of large, crowded immunoblasts with rounded nuclear contours and conspicuous central nucleoli (H&E, ×400). (*C*) Lymphoid cells express CD20 (×10), (*D*) Ki-67 (×10), (*E*) BCL2 (×10), and (*F*) MUM1 (×10; [*inset*] ×400).

Chromosomal breaks in BCL2, BCL6, and MYC are also common[46] as well as MYD88 mutations.[47–49] IgH rearrangements are present in pcDLBCL, although demonstration of clonality is not necessary for diagnosis.

Prognosis

A diagnosis of pcDLBCL is associated with a 5-year disease-specific survival of 50% to 70%. Negative prognostic indicators include location on the leg, multiple lesions, and age greater than 75 years. Patients with leg location have a mean 5-year disease-specific survival of 43% compared with 77% for others.[43] Notable factors not associated with negative impact on survival include gender, baseline performance status, serum LDH, and duration of lesions.[43,50]

Staging

NCCN guidelines include staging for all cutaneous DLBCLs. Secondary cutaneous DLBCL occurs in 7% to 10% of patients with systemic DLBCL and, therefore, is more common than pcDLBCL.[51,52] Staging includes CBC with differential, comprehensive metabolic panel, CT of the chest/abdomen/pelvis, bone marrow biopsy, PET-CT, and peripheral blood flow cytometry.[38] Testicular ultrasound is recommended for male patients with new cutaneous DLBCL given secondary cutaneous testicular DLBCL demonstrates similar presentation and pathology.[53]

Treatment

Standard treatment of pcDLBCL is based on intravenous rituximab and combination chemotherapy. Many patients with pcDLBCL are elderly and frail, making them poor candidates for chemotherapy.[43,54–56] Patients treated with a combination of chemotherapy and radiation may have a better clinical outcome than patients treated with chemotherapy alone.[57,58] A combination of multiagent chemotherapy and rituximab has been shown to have a 60% to 90% response rate and a 3-year disease-specific survival rate of 80% to 90%.[24,55,59] Unfortunately, despite chemotherapy and radiation, relapses and systemic spread are common.[40,43]

INTRAVASCULAR LARGE B-CELL LYMPHOMA

IVLBCL is a rare, aggressive, systemic non-Hodgkin lymphoma primarily diagnosed via skin biopsy. It typically affects older individuals (median age 67–70, range 13–90 years old) with poor performance status[60–63] and approximately two-thirds of patients die within 5 years.[62,64]

IVLBCL presents with proliferation of neoplastic cells in small vessel lumens. This is likely due to abnormalities in cell homing and transvascular migration.[60,62] The 2 clinical phenotypes for IVLBCL include Asian (hemophagocytic syndrome and hemophagocytic lymphohistiocytosis) and Western (cutaneous and central nervous system [CNS] involvement).[64,65]

Clinical Presentation

Cutaneous findings occur in approximately half of patients with Western IVLBCL and include maculopapular eruption, nodules, violaceous plaques, purpura, ulcers, peau d'orange changes, or cellulitis-like infiltration.[61,62,64] Distribution of involved vessels and capillary beds determines symptoms. Patients generally present with constitutional symptoms and patients with CNS involvement may demonstrate deficits in the sensory and motor nervous systems, seizures, vision loss, and altered levels of consciousness.[62,65]

Histopathology and Immunohistochemistry

IVLBCL consists of B cells distending small to medium-sized blood vessels in the dermis. Although the cells are usually large, a small cell variant has been reported in extracutaneous sites.[66] IVLBCL rarely involves the subcutis and can masquerade as panniculitis.[67] Vascular injury and involvement of adjacent dermal interstitia are exceptional findings; therefore, this disease is easily overlooked on biopsies when clinical suspicion is lacking. The lesional cells have a variable immunophenotype with BCL2 and MUM1 expression reported in most cases and variability in CD5, CD10, and BCL6 staining.[65] IgH gene rearrangement studies can help detect clonality when lymphoma is suspected histologically. A subset of IVLBCL harbor *MYD88* and *CD79b* mutations.[68]

Staging

Diagnosis is often delayed due to the heterogeneous nature of presentation and need for multiple skin or bone marrow biopsies to confirm diagnosis.[64] Imaging generally is not helpful given lack of FDG avidity of skin[63] and neuroimaging findings are nonspecific. It is believed that up to half of diagnoses are made postmortem.[60,61]

Prognosis

Both Western and Asian IVLBCLs have poor prognoses, with a mean 3-year survival of approximately 30% and median survival of 5 months.[61] Patients with cutaneous-only disease have a better prognosis.[62] Poor performance status, advanced disease, elevated serum LDH, and B symptoms are negative prognostic indicators.[65] Patients with IVLBCL respond poorly to multiagent chemotherapy,[60] but the inclusion of rituximab with other chemotherapy agents has improved survival substantially.[64] Stem cell transplant is an option for young patients with adequate performance status.[62]

REFERENCES

1. Willemze R, Kerl H, Sterry W, et al. EORTC classification for primary cutaneous lymphomas: a proposal from the Cutaneous Lymphoma Study Group of the European Organization for Research and Treatment of Cancer. Blood 1997;90(1): 354–71. Available at: http://www.ncbi.nlm.nih.gov/pubmed/9207472.

2. Bradford PT, Devesa SS, Anderson WF, et al. Cutaneous lymphoma incidence patterns in the United States: a population-based study of 3884 cases. Blood 2009;113(21):5064–73.

3. Swerdlow SH. WHO classification of tumors of haematopoietic and lymphoid tissues. Lyon: IARC; 2017.

4. Swerdlow SH, Campo E, Pileri SA, et al. The 2016 revision of the World Health Organization classification of lymphoid neoplasms. Blood 2016;127(20):2375–90.

5. Isaacson P, Chott A, Nakamura S, et al. Extranodal marginal zone lymphoma of mucosa-associated lymphoid tissue (MALT lymphoma). In: Swerdlow SH, Campo E, Harris NL, et al, editors. WHO classification of tumors of haematopoietic and lymphoid tissues. 4th edition. Lyon (France): International Agency for Research On Cancer; 2008. p. 214–7.

6. Hoefnagel J, Vermeer MH, Jansen PM, et al. Primary cutaneous marginal zone B-cell lymphoma: Clinical and theraputic features in 50 cases. Arch Dermatol 2005;141:1139–45.

7. Dalle S, Thomas L, Balme B, et al. Primary cutaneous marginal zone lymphoma. Crit Rev Oncol Hematol 2010;74:156–62.

8. Cerroni L, Signoretti S, Höfler G, et al. Primary cutaneous marginal zone B-cell lymphoma: a recently described entity of low-grade malignant cutaneous B-cell lymphoma. Am J Surg Pathol 1997;21(11):1307–15.

9. Amitay-Laish I, Tavallaee M, Kim J, et al. Paediatric primary cutaneous marginal zone B-cell lymphoma: does it differ from its adult counterpart? Br J Dermatol 2017;176(4):1010–20.

10. Servitje O, Gallardo F, Estrach T, et al. Clinical and Laboratory Investigations Primary cutaneous marginal zone B-cell lymphoma: a clinical, histopathological, immunophenotypic and molecular genetic study of 22 cases. Br J Dermatol 2002; 147:1147–58.

11. Baldassano MF, Bailey EM, Ferry JA, et al. Cutaneous lymphoid hyperplasia and cutaneous marginal zone lymphoma: comparison of morphologic and immunophenotypic features. Am J Surg Pathol 1999;23(1):88–96.

12. van Maldegem F, van Dijk R, Wormhoudt TAM, et al. The majority of cutaneous marginal zone B-cell lymphomas expresses class-switched immunoglobulins and develops in a T-helper type 2 inflammatory environment. Blood 2008;112: 3355–61.

13. Edinger JT, Kant JA, Swerdlow SH. Cutaneous marginal zone lymphomas have distinctive features and include 2 subsets. Am J Surg Pathol 2010;34(12): 1830–41.

14. Tsukamoto N, Kojima M, Uchiyama T, et al. Primary cutaneous CD5+ marginal zone B-cell lymphoma resembling the plasma cell variant of Castleman's disease. APMIS 2007;115(12):1426–31.

15. Magro CM, Yang A, Fraga G. Blastic marginal zone lymphoma: a clinical and pathological study of 8 cases and review of the literature. Am J Dermatopathol 2013;35(3):319–26.

16. Schafernak KT, Variakojis D, Goolsby CL, et al. Clonality assessment of cutaneous B-cell lymphoid proliferations: a comparison of flow cytometry immunophenotyping, molecular studies, and immunohistochemistry/in situ hybridization and review of the literature. Am J Dermatopathol 2014;36(10):781–95.

17. Geyer JT, Ferry JA, Longtine JA, et al. Characteristics of cutaneous marginal zone lymphomas with marked plasmacytic differentiation and a T cell-rich background. Am J Clin Pathol 2010;133:59–69.

18. Streubel B, Simonitsch-Klupp I, Müllauer L, et al. Variable frequencies of MALT lymphoma-associated genetic aberrations in MALT lymphomas of different sites. Leukemia 2004;18(10):1722–6.

19. Guitart J, Deonizio J, Bloom T, et al. High incidence of gastrointestinal tract disorders and autoimmunity in primary cutaneous marginal zone B-cell lymphomas. JAMA Dermatol 2014;150(4):412–8.

20. Gerami P, Wickless SC, Rosen S, et al. Applying the new TNM classification system for primary cutaneous lymphomas other than mycosis fungoides and Sézary syndrome in primary cutaneous marginal zone lymphoma. J Am Acad Dermatol 2008;59:245–54.

21. Hatem J, Schrank-Hacker AM, Watt CD, et al. Marginal zone lymphoma-derived interfollicular diffuse large B-cell lymphoma harboring 20q12 chromosomal deletion and missense mutation of BIRC3 gene: a case report. Diagn Pathol 2016; 11(1):137.

22. Zinzani PL, Quaglino P, Pimpinelli N, et al. Prognostic factors in primary cutaneous B-cell lymphoma: the Italian Study Group for Cutaneous Lymphomas. J Clin Oncol 2006;24:1376–82.

23. Willemze R, Swerdlow SH, Harris NL, et al. Primary cutaneous follicle centre lymphoma. In: Swerdlow SH, Campo E, Harris NL, et al, editors. WHO Classification of tumors of haematopoietic and lymphoid tissues. 4th edition. Lyon (France): International Agency for Research On Cancer; 2008. p. 227–8.

24. Hamilton SN, Wai ES, Tan K, et al. Treatment and outcomes in patients with primary cutaneous B-cell lymphoma: the BC Cancer Agency experience. Int J Radiat Oncol Biol Phys 2013;87(4):719–25.

25. Senff NJ, Hoefnagel JJ, Jansen PM, et al. Reclassification of 300 primary cutaneous B-Cell lymphomas according to the new WHO-EORTC classification for cutaneous lymphomas: comparison with previous classifications and identification of prognostic markers. J Clin Oncol 2007;25(12):1581–7.

26. Swerdlow SH, Quintanilla-Martinez L, Willemze R, et al. Cutaneous B-cell lymphoproliferative disorders: report of the 2011 Society for Hematopathology/European Association for Haematopathology workshop. Am J Clin Pathol 2013;139(4): 515–35.

27. Gulia A, Saggini A, Wiesner T, et al. Clinicopathologic features of early lesions of primary cutaneous follicle center lymphoma, diffuse type: implications for early diagnosis and treatment. J Am Acad Dermatol 2011;65(5):991–1000.

28. Massone C, Chott A, Metze D, et al. Subcutaneous, Blastic Natural Killer (NK), NK/T-cell, and other cytotoxic lymphomas of the skin: a morphologic, immunophenotypic, and molecular study of 50 patients. Am J Surg Pathol 2004;28(6): 719–35.

29. Aldarweesh FA, Treaba DO. Primary cutaneous follicle centre lymphoma with hodgkin and reed-sternberg like cells: a case report and review of the literature. Case Rep Hematol 2017;2017:9549428.

30. Ries S, Barr R, LeBoit P, et al. Cutaneous sarcomatoid B-cell lymphoma. Am J Dermatopathol 2007;29(1):96–8.

31. Cerroni L, El-Shabrawi-Caelen L, Fink-Puches R, et al. Cutaneous spindle-cell B-cell lymphoma: a morphologic variant of cutaneous large B-cell lymphoma. Am J Dermatopathol 2000;22(4):299–304. Available at: http://www.ncbi.nlm.nih.gov/pubmed/10949453.

32. Charli-Joseph Y, Cerroni L, LeBoit PE. Cutaneous spindle-cell B-cell Lymphomas: most are neoplasms of follicular center cell origin. Am J Surg Pathol 2015;39(6): 737–43. https://doi.org/10.1097/PAS.0000000000000388.

33. Verdanet E, Dereure O, René C, et al. Diagnostic value of STMN1, LMO2, HGAL, AID expression and 1p36 chromosomal abnormalities in primary cutaneous B cell lymphomas. Histopathology 2017;71(4):648–60.

34. Szablewski V, Ingen-Housz-Oro S, Baia M, et al. Primary cutaneous follicle center lymphomas expressing BCL2 protein frequently harbor BCL2 gene break and may present 1p36 deletion: a study of 20 cases. Am J Surg Pathol 2016;40(1): 127–36.

35. Koens L, Vermeer MH, Willemze R, et al. IgM expression on paraffin sections distinguishes primary cutaneous large B-cell lymphoma, leg type from primary cutaneous follicle center lymphoma. Am J Surg Pathol 2010;34(7):1043–8.

36. Robson A, Shukur Z, Ally M, et al. Immunocytochemical p63 expression discriminates between primary cutaneous follicle centre cell and diffuse large B cell lymphoma-leg type, and is of the TAp63 isoform. Histopathology 2016;69(1): 11–9.

37. Plaza JA, Kacerovska D, Sangueza M, et al. Can cutaneous low-grade B-cell lymphoma transform into primary cutaneous diffuse large B-cell lymphoma? An

immunohistochemical study of 82 cases. Am J Dermatopathol 2014;36(6): 478–82.

38. NCCN Guidelines for Primary Cutaneous B-cell Lymphomas. Available at: https:// www.nccn.org/professionals/physician_gls/pdf/pcbcl.pdf. Accessed May 28, 2018.

39. Goyal A, Carter JB, Pashtan I, et al. Very low-dose versus standard dose radiation therapy for indolent primary cutaneous B cell lymphomas: a retrospective study. J Am Acad Dermatol 2018;78(2):408–10.

40. Meijer CJLM, Vergier B, Duncan LM, et al. Primary cutaneous DLBCL, leg type. In: Swerdlow SH, Campo E, Harris NL, et al, editors. WHO classification of tumors of haematopoietic and lymphoid tissues. 4th edition. Lyon (France): International Agency for Research on Cancer; 2008. p. 242.

41. Paulli M, Viglio A, Vivenza D, et al. Primary cutaneous large B-cell lymphoma of the leg: histogenetic analysis of a controversial clinicopathologic entity. Hum Pathol 2002;33(9):937–43.

42. Vermeer MH, Geelen F, van Haselen CW, et al. Primary cutaneous large B-cell lymphoma of the leg. Arch Dermatol 1996;132:1304–8.

43. Grange F, Beylot-Barry M, Courville P, et al. Primary cutaneous diffuse large B-cell lymphoma, leg type. Arch Dermatol 2007;143(9):1144–50.

44. Kodama K, Massone C, Chott A, et al. Primary cutaneous large B-cell lymphomas: clinicopathologic features, classification, and prognostic factors in a large series of patients. Blood 2005;106(7):2491–7.

45. Senff NJ, Zoutman WH, Vermeer MH, et al. Fine-mapping chromosomal loss at 9p21: correlation with prognosis in primary cutaneous diffuse large B-cell lymphoma, leg type. J Invest Dermatol 2009;129(5):1149–55.

46. Menguy S, Frison E, Prochazkova-Carlotti M, et al. Double-hit or dual expression of MYC and BCL2 in primary cutaneous large B-cell lymphomas. Mod Pathol 2018. https://doi.org/10.1038/s41379-018-0041-7.

47. Mareschal S, Pham-Ledard A, Viailly PJ, et al. Identification of somatic mutations in primary cutaneous diffuse large B-cell lymphoma, leg type by massive parallel sequencing. J Invest Dermatol 2017;137(9):1984–94.

48. Pham-Ledard A, Cappellen D, Martinez F, et al. MYD88 somatic mutation is a genetic feature of primary cutaneous diffuse large B-cell lymphoma, leg type. J Invest Dermatol 2012;132(8):2118–20.

49. Menguy S, Gros A, Pham-Ledard A, et al. MYD88 somatic mutation is a diagnostic criterion in primary cutaneous large B-cell lymphoma. J Invest Dermatol 2016;136(8):1741–4.

50. Kramer MH, Hermans J, Wijburg E, et al. Clinical relevance of BCL2, BCL6, and MYC rearrangements in diffuse large B-cell lymphoma. Blood 1998;92(9): 3152–62.

51. Sterry W, Kruger GR, Steigelder G-K. Skin involvement in malignant B-cell lymphomas. J Dermatol Surg Oncol 1984;10(4):276–7.

52. Morton LM, Wang SS, Devesa SS, et al. Lymphoma incidence patterns by WHO subtype in the United States, 1992-2001. Blood 2006;107(1):265–76.

53. Muniesa C, Pujol RM, Estrach MT, et al. Primary cutaneous diffuse large B-cell lymphoma, leg type and secondary cutaneous involvement by testicular B-cell lymphoma share identical clinicopathological and immunophenotypical features. J Am Acad Dermatol 2012;66(4):650–4.

54. Brogan BL, Zic JA, Kinney MC, et al. Large B-cell lymphoma of the leg: clinical and pathologic characteristics in a north american series. J Am Acad Dermatol 2003;49(2):223–8.

55. Grange F, Maubec E, Bagot M, et al. Treatment of cutaneous B-cell lymphoma, leg type, with age-adapted combinations of chemotherapies and rituximab. Arch Dermatol 2009;145(3):329–30.
56. Senff NJ, Noordijk EM, Kim YH, et al. European Organization for Research and Treatment of Cancer and International Society for Cutaneous Lymphoma consensus recommendations for the management of cutaneous B-cell lymphomas. Blood 2008;112(5):1600–9.
57. Persky DO, Unger JM, Spier CM, et al. Phase II study of rituximab plus three cycles of CHOP and involved-field radiotherapy for patients with limited-stage aggressive B-cell lymphoma: Southwest Oncology Group study 0014. J Clin Oncol 2008;26(14):2258–63.
58. Miller TP, Dahlberg S, Cassady JR, et al. Chemotherapy alone compared with chemotherapy plus radiotherapy for localized intermediate- and high-grade non-Hodgkin's lymphoma. N Engl J Med 1998;339(1):21–6.
59. Posada-Garcia C, Florez A, Pardavila R, et al. Primary cutaneous large B-cell lymphoma, leg type, successfully treated with rituximab plus chemotherapy. Eur J Dermatol 2009;19(4):393–4.
60. Nakamura S, Ponzoni M, Campo E. Intravascular large B-cell lymphoma. In: Swerdlow SH, Campo E, Harris NL, et al, editors. WHO classification of tumors of haematopoietic and lymphoid tissues. Lyon (France): International Agency for Research On Cancer; 2008. p. 252–3.
61. Ferreri AJM, Campo E, Seymour JF, et al. Intravascular lymphoma: clinical presentation, natural history, management and prognostic factors in a series of 38 cases, with special emphasis on the "cutaneous variant". Br J Haematol 2004; 127(2):173–83.
62. Orwat DE, Batalis NI. Intravascular large B-cell lymphoma. Arch Pathol Lab Med 2012;136(3):333–8.
63. Ponzoni M, Ferreri AJM, Campo E, et al. Definition, diagnosis, and management of intravascular large B-cell lymphoma: proposals and perspectives from an international consensus meeting. J Clin Oncol 2007;25(21):3168–73.
64. Shimada K, Kinoshita T, Naoe T, et al. Presentation and management of intravascular large B-cell lymphoma. Lancet Oncol 2009;10(9):895–902.
65. Murase T, Yamaguchi M, Suzuki R, et al. Intravascular large B-cell lymphoma (IVLBCL): a clinicopathologic study of 96 cases with special reference to the immunophenotypic heterogeneity of CD5. Blood 2007;109(2):478–85.
66. Rahmani M, Halene S, Xu ML. Small cell variant of intravascular large B-cell lymphoma: highlighting a potentially fatal and easily missed diagnosis. Biomed Res Int 2018;2018:9413015.
67. Phoon YW, Lin X, Thirumoorthy T, et al. Intravascular large B-cell lymphoma presenting as panniculitis clinically: a case report. Singapore Med J 2018;59(3): 163–4.
68. Schrader AMR, Jansen PM, Willemze R, et al. High prevalence of MYD88 and CD79B mutations in intravascular large B-cell lymphoma. Blood 2018;131(18): 2086–9.

Cutaneous Involvement of Hematologic Malignancies

Nancy Kaddis, MD, MPH[a], David Fisher, MD[b], Eric D. Jacobsen, MD[b],*

KEYWORDS

- Secondary cutaneous lymphoma • Histiocyte disorders
- Langerhans cell histiocytosis (LCH) • Rosai-Dorfman disease (RDD)

KEY POINTS

- A broad array of hematologic malignancies can manifest with primary or secondary cutaneous involvement; the authors discuss pathologic and clinical presentations of several of these diseases: secondary cutaneous lymphomas and histiocyte disorders involving the skin.
- Secondary cutaneous lymphoma is defined as infiltration of lymphoma cells in the skin as a result of disseminated systemic T-cell/natural killer (NK)-cell and B-cell lymphomas.
- Histiocytic disorders are well known to involve the skin, and 2 common histiocytic disorders with cutaneous manifestations are reviewed.

SECONDARY CUTANEOUS INVOLVEMENT WITH LYMPHOMA

Cutaneous manifestations of hematologic malignancies include paraneoplastic dermatoses, secondary infiltration of the skin in the setting of systemic disease, or primary cutaneous malignancies, such as primary cutaneous lymphomas (PCLs). PCLs, such as mycosis fungoides, Sézary syndrome, and primary cutaneous B-cell lymphomas, are generally confined to the skin (and occasionally blood) at diagnosis with no evidence of extracutaneous involvement at the time of presentation (although this can occur later in the illness). PCLs account for 19% of extranodal non-Hodgkin lymphomas[1] and have distinct clinical behavior, prognosis, and treatment paradigms from histologically similar systemic lymphomas, including those with secondary skin involvement.

In this section, the authors focus on secondary cutaneous lymphomas (SCLs), which are defined as skin lesions that developed concurrently or after a diagnosis

Disclosure Statement: No commercial or financial conflicts of interest or any funding sources exist for any of the authors.
[a] Department of Hematology and Oncology, Dana-Farber Cancer Institute at St Elizabeth's Medical Center, 736 Cambridge Street, Brighton, MA 02135, USA; [b] Lymphoma Clinic, Dana-Farber Cancer Institute, 450 Brookline Avenue, Boston, MA 02215, USA
* Corresponding author.
E-mail address: Eric_Jacobsen@dfci.harvard.edu

Hematol Oncol Clin N Am 33 (2019) 163–172
https://doi.org/10.1016/j.hoc.2018.08.005
0889-8588/19/© 2018 Elsevier Inc. All rights reserved.

of systemic lymphoma. The relative incidence, clinical features, biology, and prognoses of SCLs remain poorly understood although SCLs constitute 20% to 50% of cutaneous lymphomas. Following is a review of studies that described the clinical characteristics and outcomes of large cohorts of SCL patients.

One retrospective cohort study of 106 patients with SCL divided cases by cell lineage: T-cell/natural killer (NK)-cell versus B-cell lineages. In this cohort, 56% were found to be mature T-cell/NK-cell lymphomas, 35% were mature B-cell lymphomas, 8% were immature hematopoietic malignancies and 1% were Hodgkin lymphoma.[2] Demographics between the 2 lineages differed, with patients with B-cell lymphoma presenting at a significantly older age versus those with T-cell/NK-cell lineage lymphoma; gender ratio did not differ significantly between the 2 subtypes. T-cell/NK-cell lymphoma more often had disseminated involvement with multiple skin lesions than those of B-cell lineage. Lymph node involvement was the most common primary tumor site in both subtypes though extranodal involvement because a primary site was more common with NK-cell/T-cell lymphomas. Other clinical characteristics, including lactate dehydrogenase (LDH), stage, presence of lymphadenopathy, and visceral involvement, did not differ between the T-cell/NK-cell and B-cell lineages. Bone marrow involvement, however, was much more common in T-cell/NK-cell lineage lymphoma than in B-cell lineage lymphoma cases.[2]

The appearance of the skin lesions also differed between the 2 cell lineages. Patients with T-cell/NK-cell lymphomas were more likely to have macular patches than patients with B-cell lymphoma. Ulcerations were noted in 25% of patients with NK-cell/T-cell lymphoma and in only 3% of those with B-cell lymphoma (**Fig. 1**). The mean time of cutaneous dissemination was 10.3 months after the initial diagnosis of the primary systemic disease and did not differ based on the cell lineage.[2]

Overall survival (OS) did not differ statistically based on the lineage of the lymphoma (5-year OS of the T-cell/NK-cell lymphoma lineage was 29% whereas that of the B-cell lymphoma lineage was 33%; $P = .468$). Patients who developed skin lesions within 6 months of initial diagnosis, however, had shorter median OS of 13 months than patients who developed cutaneous dissemination 6 or more months after initial diagnosis who had a median OS of 38 months ($P<.001$). Those with disseminated skin lesions had a poorer median OS of 16 months compared with a median OS of 37 months in

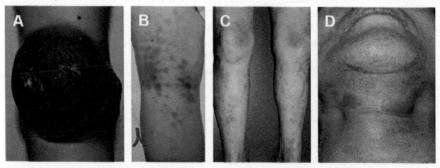

Fig. 1. Cutaneous manifestations of SCLs. (*A*) A solitary ulcerated nodule on the lower extremity in extranodal NK-cell/T-cell lymphoma. (*B*) Multiple macular patches on the arm in angioimmunoblastic T-cell lymphoma. (*C*) Multiple erythematous to brownish macules and papules on the legs in peripheral T-cell lymphoma. (*D*) Multiple subcutaneous nodules on the neck in DLBCL. (*From* Lee WJ, Won KH, Won CH, et al. Secondary cutaneous lymphoma: comparative clinical features and survival outcome analysis of 106 cases according to lymphoma cell lineage. Br J Dermatol 2015;173(1):134–45; with permission.)

those with localized skin lesions ($P = .028$). Additionally, patients with an elevated serum LDH at diagnosis had a median OS of 19 months and those with a normal serum LDH had a median OS of 37 months ($P = .024$). Finally, primary site of tumor was also identified as a prognostic factor with those who had lymph node involvement as a primary site of disease having a median OS of 36 months compared with 19 months for those with extranodal disease as a primary site ($P = .036$). Traditional prognostic factors in lymphomas, such as age and IPI, seem to have no prognostic relevance in SCL, although overall, outcomes of patients with SCL are significantly worse than those of patients with PCL (in 1 study 5-year survival rate of patients with SCL was 31% whereas that of PCL was 87%–93%).[3]

In a subset of these 106 patients with SCLs, 8 were identified as secondary peripheral T-cell lymphoma unspecified and had dissemination of disease involving the entire body. The clinical and histopathologic findings of these 8 patients were consistent (**Fig. 2**). None had epidermal ulcerations, epidermal spongiosis, or interface reactions. All cases of SCL expressed T-cell markers, including CD3 and CD4, and all but 2 expressed CD8. All were negative for CD56 and CD20. T-cell receptor gene rearrangements were present in all 8 cases whereas Epstein-Barr virus was negative in all cases.[3]

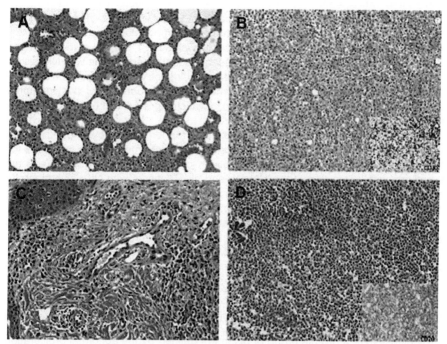

Fig. 2. Histopathologic findings in SCL. (*A*) NK-cell/T-cell lymphoma. Panniculitis: infiltration of medium-sized tumor cells with a pattern of rimming (hematoxylin-eosin [H&E] stain). (*B*) Anaplastic large cell lymphoma with sheets of CD30+ large cells containing prominent vacuoles and nucleoli (H&E stain). (*C*) Angioimmunoblastic lymphoma showing perivascular atypical lymphocytic infiltration and capillary hyperplasia (H&E stain). (*D*) DLBCL. Confluent sheets of large CD20+ tumor cells noted (H&E stain). (*From* Lee WJ, Kang HJ, Won CH, et al. Secondary cutaneous peripheral T-cell lymphoma, unspecified, with generalized benign-looking dermatitis: a possibly distinct peripheral T-cell lymphoma. Int J Dermatol 2017;56(6):617–22; with permission.)

A Dutch registry reported on 219 patients with CD30$^+$ (anaplastic) primary or SCL followed over a 15-year period (1983–1998) to examine methods of diagnosis and treatment in these patients.[4] Characteristics of skin lesions differed between the groups. SCL patients presented more frequently with papules and nodules and less frequently with tumor-type skin lesions and plaques than their counterparts with PCL. At diagnosis, none of the PCL patients had B-symptoms whereas 55% of the SCL patients did. Initial therapy differed, as was expected; 82% of SCL patients were treated with multiagent chemotherapy whereas only 8% of PCL patients received this therapy. In contrast, 48% of PCL patients received radiotherapy, 19% had excisions of their lesion, 19% had topical steroids, and 4% had psoralen–UV-A/UV-B treatment. For SCL patients, only 18% received radiotherapy and none received excision, topical steroids, or psoralen–UV-A/UV-B treatment.

Outcomes also differed between the 2 groups in this study. In comparison to patients with PCL, those with SCL had substantially lower 5-year survival rates of 24% compared with those with PCL, who had 5-year survival rates of 96%. Systemic relapse occurred in 55% of SCL patients but only 4% in PCL patients. Mortality differed as well; 5% of the PCL patients died of lymphoma compared with 73% of SCL patients.[4] Thus, it is important to avoid aggressive multiagent chemotherapy in patients with primary cutaneous CD30$^+$ lymphoproliferative disorders.

In another retrospective review of 62 patients with cutaneous lymphoma in Japan, 31 cases of PCL were compared with 31 cases of SCL. Of the SCL cases, T-cell and NK-cell lymphomas accounted for 54% and B-cell lymphomas accounted for 46%.[5] The most common subtype of T-cell lymphoma was adult T-cell leukemia lymphoma (ATLL), of which there were 9 cases. The second most common type was NK-cell/T-cell lymphoma, nasal type, followed by an equal incidence of anaplastic large cell lymphoma and blastic NK-cell lymphoma. The most common subtype of B-cell lymphoma was diffuse large B-cell lymphoma (DLBCL), of which there were 11 cases followed by follicular lymphoma (2 patients).[5]

The ages of those with T-cell and NK-cell lymphoma was lower (median age 64 years) than those with secondary B-cell lymphomas (median age 69). Male-to-female ratio was similar between the T-cell/NK-cell and the B-cell SCLs. Six of the 9 patients with ATLL died of the disease and all 5 patients with NK-cell lymphoma died within 3 years. Of the 11 patients with DLBCL, 7 died within a year of developing cutaneous disease.[5]

Although there are few data on SCL, the available studies all indicate that patients with SCL have a poor prognosis compared with patients with PCL. Differentiating PCL from SCL can be challenging and requires integration of clinical, radiographic, and pathology data. Differentiating between these 2 entities, however, is crucial for diagnostic, prognostic, and treatment purposes.

CUTANEOUS INVOLVEMENT WITH THE HISTIOCYTOSES

Histiocytoses are a diverse group of disorders defined by the abnormal proliferation and accumulation of neoplastic cells of monocyte/macrophage derivation. This article discusses 2 histiocytic disorders that commonly present with skin manifestations.

The most common of these disorders is Langerhans cell histiocytosis (LCH). The Langerhans cell (LC) is a cutaneous antigen-presenting cell that is derived from CD34$^+$ bone marrow progenitors and migrates into the epidermis. LCs are antigen-presenting cells that induce antigen-specific T-cell responses.[6] LCH is the result of over-proliferation and accumulation of LCs in tissues, which cause tissue damage partially through cytokine production. LCs stain positive for S-100, CD1a, and

Langerin (CD207); the most specific of these for LCH are CD1a and Langerin. Organelles called Birbeck granules are seen on electron microscopy in LCs but the characteristic immunophenotype and morphology have rendered electron microscopy obsolete for clinical purposes.[7]

Recurrent BRAF V600E mutations have been identified in approximately 50% to 60% of cases of LCH and in some circumstances can be found in the CD34$^+$ progenitors, thus confirming LCH as a clonal malignancy of myeloid dendritic cell derivation.[8] The BRAF protein is a member of the Raf kinase family of growth signal transduction protein kinases, which play a role in the regulation of the MAP kinase/ERKs signaling pathway.[9] Dysregulation of the RAS/RAF pathway seems to be a defining feature of LCH because patients who are BRAF wild-type frequently have ARAF, MAP2K1, or other RAS/RAF pathway mutations.[10,11]

LCH can present with unifocal (55% of cases) or multifocal (45% of cases) involvement of various organs. In 1 retrospective review of 1741 patients with LCH, the organs most involved in decreasing frequency were bone, skin, lymph nodes, liver, spleen, oral mucosa, lung, and central nervous system.[12] Multisystem disease is most commonly seen in younger children whereas unifocal disease is more common in older children and adults. Presenting symptoms in adults, in order of decreasing frequency, are skin rash, dyspnea or tachypnea, polydipsia and polyuria, bone pain, lymphadenopathy, weight loss, fever, gingival hypertrophy, ataxia, and memory problems.[10,13,14] Because a large proportion of patients with LCH have cutaneous lesions, skin biopsy can provide a mechanism for rapid and noninvasive diagnosis.

The most common skin manifestations in LCH are brown to purplish papules, although other manifestations do occur (**Fig. 3**).[15] Cutaneous lesions most often involve the scalp, face, trunk, and perineum.

Cutaneous LCH is typically treated with skin-directed therapy, including topical steroids, topical nitrogen mustard, phototherapy, and surgical curettage for unifocal disease.[16] Surgical excision may be curative in unifocal skin involvement and low dose radiation can be used for palliation.[14] Chemotherapeutic agents, such as vinblastine, cladribine, cytarabine, clofarabine, methotrexate, 6-mercaptopurine, and systemic steroids, are commonly used in multifocal LCH but rarely needed for isolated cutaneous involvement.[14,17,18]

Rosai-Dorfman disease (RDD) (or sinus histiocytosis with massive lymphadenopathy) is a non-LCH that also frequently has cutaneous and/or subcutaneous involvement. In most circumstances RDD is likely a reactive histiocytosis with a self-limited and benign course although mutations in known oncogenes have been described. Histologic examination of RDD reveals enlargement of the lymph node sinuses by large foamy histiocytosis mixed with plasma cells within a prominent capsule. Emperipolesis, the presence of intact lymphocytes and/or plasma cells within the histiocytes, is a near universal although not pathognomonic finding and tends to be more notable in lymph nodes than in skin lesions.[19]

RDD is typically S100 positive and CD1a negative, which, along with the lack of CD207 and Birbeck granules, differentiates RDD from LCH. RDD is also positive for factor XIIIa.[20] Activating KRAS and MAP2K1 mutations have been reported in approximately one-third of cases of RDD (**Fig. 4** and **Fig. 5**).[21,22]

The exact etiology and pathophysiology of RDD is not clear. There is a clear association between RDD and autoimmune diseases; in approximately 10% of cases of RDD, an underlying autoimmune disease is found.[23] The most common of these coexisting autoimmune diseases are systemic lupus erythematous, idiopathic juvenile arthritis, autoimmune hemolytic anemia, and RAS-associated autoimmune leukoproliferative disease.[24] RDD has also been associated with several malignancies, notably

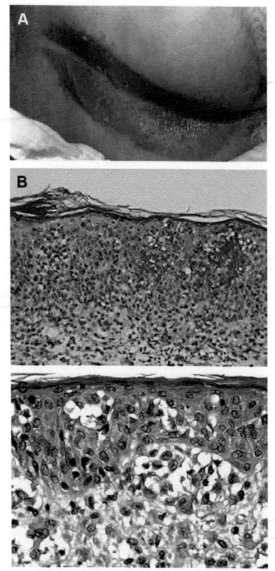

Fig. 3. Langerhans cell disease of the skin. (*A*) Presentation of Letterer-Siwe disease. A disseminated form of LCD in buttock area of a child. (*B*) Hematoxylin-eosin–stained sections of a skin biopsy show infiltrates in the dermis and prominently in the epidermis. (*C*) Cutaneous infiltrates appear oval with eosinophilic cytoplasm and an occasional nuclear groove (LCs). (*From* Newman B, Hu W, Nigro K, et al. Aggressive histiocytic disorders that can involve the skin. J Am Acad Dermatol 2007;56(2):304; with permission.)

Hodgkin and non-Hodgkin lymphomas,[25] and less often myelodysplastic syndrome[26] or postallogeneic bone marrow transplant.[27]

The characteristic patient is an otherwise healthy young man presenting with painless bilateral cervical adenopathy, polyclonal gammopathy with a reversal of the CD4/CD8 ratio and an elevated erythrocyte sedimentation rate. B-symptoms are not

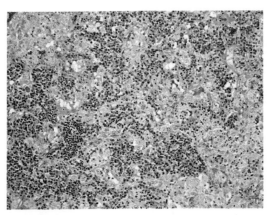

Fig. 4. Rosai-Dorfman disease. The lymph node sinuses contain sheets of large pithelioid cells with abundant pale cytoplasm. Note the numerous admixed plasma cells (hematoxylin-eosin, original magnification ×200).

uncommon at diagnosis. In addition, 43% of patients present with extranodal involvement of which the skin is the most common organ involved, followed by bone and central nervous system involvement.[28] In half of these cases, the skin is the only involved organ. Lesions can involve any area of the body and most often follow a benign course and regress spontaneously.[28]

The optimal treatment of RDD is unknown and spontaneous resolution is common. For nodal or cutaneous disease, steroids have been used with variable response.[29–32] Traditionally, for recurrent and relapsing cases, vinblastine, etoposide, methotrexate, cyclosporine, and radiation have been used with variable efficacy.[28] Targeted therapy with MEK inhibitors, such as cometinib, to block the activating RAS and MAPK pathway, are being studied in current phase II trials and have been successful in several patients with a known KRAS mutation.[33,34] Imatinib has shown variable results in treating RDD.[35,36]

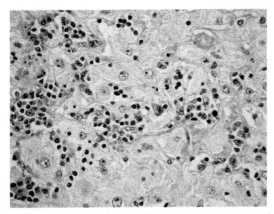

Fig. 5. Rosai-Dorfman disease. The lesional cells contain central, round nuclei with small nucleoli and voluminous pale cytoplasm. The plasma cells and lymphocytes lie within the cytoplasm of the lesional cells (emperipolesis) (hematoxylin-eosin; original magnification ×600).

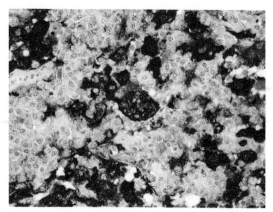

Fig. 6. Rosai-Dorfman disease. Immunohistochemistry for S100 protein is strongly positive in the lesion cells and highlights emperipolesis (cell in the center of the field) (original magnification ×600).

According to recently published consensus guidelines for RDD, when treating RDD with systemic agents, such as steroids or other drugs, evaluating for response to treatment should be done within 4 months.[37] Patients with disease localized to lymph nodes or skin have shown more favorable outcomes, whereas patients with extranodal disease, in particular those with renal, hepatic, or thoracic involvement, have poorer outcomes. More aggressive treatments, such as systemic chemotherapy or clinical trials, may be indicated in these cases **(Fig. 6)**.[37]

SUMMARY

A variety of hematologic malignancies can involve the skin. Differentiating primary from secondary cutaneous involvement can have critical therapeutic and prognostic implications, particularly in lymphoma. Currently there is a dearth of data regarding the etiology, prognosis, and optimal treatment of patients with secondary skin involvement with various hematologic malignancies; multidisciplinary collaboration between medical oncology and dermatology is critical in optimally managing these patients.

REFERENCES

1. Groves FD, Linet MS, Travis LB, et al. Cancer surveillance series: non-Hodgkin's lymphoma incidence by histologic subtype in the United States from 1978 through 1995. J Natl Cancer Inst 2000;92(15):1240–51.

2. Lee WJ, Won KH, Won CH, et al. Secondary cutaneous lymphoma: comparative clinical features and survival outcome analysis of 106 cases according to lymphoma cell lineage. Br J Dermatol 2015;173(1):134–45.

3. Lee WJ, Kang HJ, Won CH, et al. Secondary cutaneous peripheral T-cell lymphoma, unspecified, with generalized benign-looking dermatitis: a possibly distinct peripheral T-cell lymphoma. Int J Dermatol 2017;56(6):617–22.

4. Bekkenk MW, Geelen FA, van Voorst Vader PC, et al. Primary and secondary cutaneous CD30(+) lymphoproliferative disorders: a report from the Dutch Cutaneous Lymphoma Group on the long-term follow-up data of 219 patients and guidelines for diagnosis and treatment. Blood 2000;95(12):3653–61.

5. Yasukawa K, Kato N, Kodama K, et al. The spectrum of cutaneous lymphomas in Japan: a study of 62 cases based on the World Health Organization Classification. J Cutan Pathol 2006;33(7):487–91.

6. Romani N, Holzmann S, Tripp CH, et al. Langerhans cells - dendritic cells of the epidermis [review]. APMIS 2003;111(7–8):725–40.

7. Mazal PR, Hainfellner JA, Preiser J, et al. Langerhans cell histiocytosis of the hypothalamus: diagnostic value of immunohistochemistry. Clin Neuropathol 1996; 15(2):87–91.

8. Grois N, Pötschger U, Prosch H, et al, DALHX- and LCH I and II Study Committee. Risk factors for diabetes insipidus in langerhans cell histiocytosis. Pediatr Blood Cancer 2006;46(2):228–33.

9. Badalian-Very G, Vergilio JA, Degar BA, et al. Recurrent BRAF mutations in Langerhans cell histiocytosis. Blood 2010;116(11):1919–23.

10. Berres ML, Lim KP, Peters T, et al. BRAF-V600E expression in precursor versus differentiated dendritic cells defines clinically distinct LCH risk groups. J Exp Med 2014;211(4):669–83.

11. Chakraborty R, Hampton OA, Shen X, et al. Mutually exclusive recurrent somatic mutations in MAP2K1 and BRAF support a central role for ERK activation in LCH pathogenesis. Blood 2014;124(19):3007–15.

12. Baumgartner I, von Hochstetter A, Baumert B, et al. Langerhans'-cell histiocytosis in adults. Med Pediatr Oncol 1997;28(1):9–14.

13. Islinger RB, Kuklo TR, Owens BD, et al. Langerhans' cell histiocytosis in patients older than 21 years. Clin Orthop Relat Res 2000;(379):231–5.

14. Götz G, Fichter J. Langerhans'-cell histiocytosis in 58 adults. Eur J Med Res 2004;9(11):510–4.

15. Newman B, Hu W, Nigro K, et al. Aggressive histiocytic disorders that can involve the skin [review]. J Am Acad Dermatol 2007;56(2):302–16.

16. Duan MH, Han X, Li J, et al. Comparison of vindesine and prednisone and cyclophosphamide, etoposide, vindesine, and prednisone as first-line treatment for adult Langerhans cell histiocytosis: a single-center retrospective study. Leuk Res 2016;42:43–6.

17. Girschikofsky M, Arico M, Castillo D, et al. Management of adult patients with Langerhans cell histiocytosis: recommendations from an expert panel on behalf of Euro-Histio-Net [review]. Orphanet J Rare Dis 2013;8:72.

18. Egeler RM, Annels NE, Hogendoorn PC. Langerhans cell histiocytosis: a pathologic combination of oncogenesis and immune dysregulation. Pediatr Blood Cancer 2004;42(5):401–3.

19. Chou TC, Tsai KB, Lee CH. Emperipolesis is not pathognomonic for Rosai-Dorfman disease: rhinoscleroma mimicking Rosai-Dorfman disease, a clinical series. J Am Acad Dermatol 2013;69(6):1066–7.

20. Ortonne N, Fillet AM, Kosuge H, et al. Cutaneous Destombes-Rosai-Dorfman disease: absence of detection of HHV-6 and HHV-8 in skin. J Cutan Pathol 2002; 29(2):113–8.

21. Diamond EL, Durham BH, Haroche J, et al. Diverse and targetable kinase alterations drive histiocytic neoplasms. Cancer Discov 2016;6(2):154–65.

22. Garces S, Medeiros LJ, Patel KP, et al. Mutually exclusive recurrent KRAS and MAP2K1 mutations in Rosai-Dorfman disease. Mod Pathol 2017;30(10):1367–77.

23. Foucar E, Rosai J, Dorfman R. Sinus histiocytosis with massive lymphadenopathy (Rosai-Dorfman disease): review of the entity [review]. Semin Diagn Pathol 1990; 7(1):19–73.

24. Vaiselbuh SR, Bryceson YT, Allen CE, et al. Updates on histiocytic disorders. Pediatr Blood Cancer 2014;61(7):1329–35.
25. Ragotte RJ, Dhanrajani A, Pleydell-Pearce J, et al. The importance of considering monogenic causes of autoimmunity: a somatic mutation in KRAS causing pediatric Rosai-Dorfman syndrome and systemic lupus erythematosus. Clin Immunol 2017;175:143–6.
26. Long E, Lassalle S, Cheikh-Rouhou R, et al. Intestinal occlusion caused by Rosai-Dorfman disease mimicking colonic diverticulitis. Pathol Res Pract 2007;203(4):233–7.
27. Ambati S, Chamyan G, Restrepo R, et al. Rosai-Dorfman disease following bone marrow transplantation for pre-B cell acute lymphoblastic leukemia. Pediatr Blood Cancer 2008;51(3):433–5.
28. Pulsoni A, Anghel G, Falcucci P, et al. Treatment of sinus histiocytosis with massive lymphadenopathy (Rosai-Dorfman disease): report of a case and literature review [review]. Am J Hematol 2002;69(1):67–71.
29. Adeleye AO, Amir G, Fraifeld S, et al. Diagnosis and management of Rosai-Dorfman disease involving the central nervous system [review]. Neurol Res 2010;32(6):572–8.
30. Petrushkin H, Salisbury J, O'Sullivan E. Intralesional steroid for orbital manifestations of Rosai-Dorfman disease. Clin Exp Ophthalmol 2015;43(5):483–5.
31. Ottaviano G, Doro D, Marioni G, et al. Extranodal Rosai-Dorfman disease: involvement of eye, nose and trachea. Acta Otolaryngol 2006;126(6):657–60.
32. Sakallioglu O, Gok F, Kalman S, et al. Minimal change nephropathy in a 7-year-old boy with Rosai-Dorfman disease. J Nephrol 2006;19(2):211–4.
33. Diamond EL, Durham BH, Dogan A, et al. Phase 2 trial of single-agent cometinib for adults with histiocytic disorders: preliminary results. Presented at the Erdheim Chester Global Alliance Medical Symposium, New York, September 12–17, 2016. [abstract: 257].
34. Jacobsen E, Shanmugam V, Jagannathan J. Rosai-Dorfman disease with activating KRAS Mutation - response to cobimetinib. N Engl J Med 2017;377(24):2398–9.
35. Utikal J, Ugurel S, Kurzen H, et al. Imatinib as a treatment option for systemic non-Langerhans cell histiocytoses. Arch Dermatol 2007;143(6):736–40.
36. Gebhardt C, Averbeck M, Paasch U, et al. A case of cutaneous Rosai-Dorfman disease refractory to imatinib therapy. Arch Dermatol 2009;145(5):571–4.
37. Abla O, Jacobsen E, Picarsic J, et al. Consensus recommendations for the diagnosis and clinical management of Rosai-Dorfman-Destombes disease [review]. Blood 2018;131(26):2877–90.

Cutaneous Metastasis

John D. Strickley, BS[a,b], Alfred Bennett Jenson, MS, MD[a],
Jae Yeon Jung, MD, PhD[a,c,d],*

KEYWORDS

- Metastasis • Cutaneous metastases • Skin • Melanoma • Breast cancer
- Dermatology • Oncology

KEY POINTS

- Cutaneous metastases may be the first sign of an internal malignancy and in general portend a poor prognosis. The incidence is increasing due to improved survival of patients with cancer as a whole.
- Although most cutaneous metastases will classically appear as a dermal nodule, there have been a wide range of clinical appearances reported, many of which are described in this article.
- Breast cancer and melanoma are the most common cancers to spread to/within the skin, but other malignancies (such as lung, colon, renal, head and neck, and hematologic) are frequently implicated.
- Systemic chemotherapeutics targeting the primary tumor appear to be the standard of care, but skin-directed therapies and immunotherapies have shown efficacy.

INTRODUCTION

Cutaneous metastasis accounts for only 2% of all skin cancers,[1] but incidence is increasing due to improved survival of patients with cancer as a whole.[2] The importance of prompt recognition of a cutaneous metastasis is highlighted by the fact that it can be the first clinical sign of a new or recurrent malignancy. Understanding epidemiology and the spectrum of clinical presentations improves diagnostic accuracy, allowing for prompt biopsy and initiation of the appropriate therapy. In the setting

Disclosure Statement: J.Y. Jung - Regeneron: Principal investigator, Consultant; Merck: Principal investigator; Iderra: Principal investigator; Adgero: Consultant; Amgen: Consultant, Speaker.
[a] James Graham Brown Cancer Center, University of Louisville School of Medicine, 529 S. Jackson Street, Louisville, KY 40202, USA; [b] Department of Dermatology, Center for Cancer Immunology and Cutaneous Biology Research Center, MGH Cancer Center, Massachusetts General Hospital, Harvard Medical School, Boston, MA 02129, USA; [c] Division of Dermatology, University of Louisville School of Medicine, 3810 Springhurst Boulevard, Suite. 200, Louisville, KY 40241, USA; [d] Onco-Dermatology Program, Norton Cancer Institute, 676 South Floyd Street, Suite 200, Louisville, KY 40202, USA
* Corresponding author. 676 South Floyd Street, Suite 200, Louisville, KY 40202.
E-mail address: Jae.jung@nortonhealthcare.org

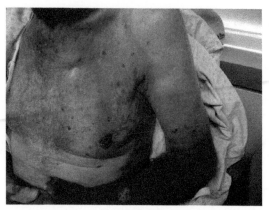

Fig. 1. Distant cutaneous metastases from melanoma are considered clinically stage IV disease. Also note the development of vitiligo following interferon therapy.

of melanoma and breast cancers, timely diagnosis and referral can significantly impact the patient's overall prognosis. **Figs. 1–32** highlight the scope and breadth of cutaneous metastases.

Although classically appearing as a dermal nodule (see **Fig. 1**),[2,3] the clinical appearance of cutaneous metastases can vary widely (see **Figs. 2–4**), thus clinicians must have a high index of suspicion based on various factors.[2,3] For instance, patient sex and primary cancer type are two key elements when considering this diagnosis. In 1993, a landmark study by Lookingbill and colleagues[3] reported melanoma (32.2%), lung (11.8%), and colon (11.0%) cancers account for most cases in men, whereas breast cancer (70%) accounts for the overwhelming majority of cases in women[1] (**Fig. 33**). Biopsy of suspect lesions will provide the diagnosis and typically offers the origin of malignant cells (via cytomorphology and immunohistochemistry). Life expectancy following diagnosis depends on the primary cancer type, but skin metastasis

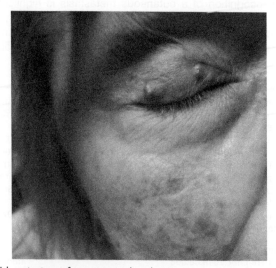

Fig. 2. Rare eyelid metastases from mucosal melanoma.

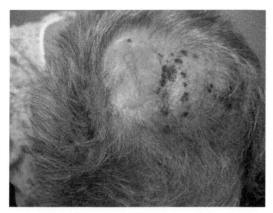

Fig. 3. Classic appearance of in-transit melanoma metastases, within 2 cm of the resected margins.

in general is associated with poor prognosis (**Fig. 34**).[3–6] Skin metastases tend to occur in the general region of the primary tumor, but cases of distant spread to unique locations, such as the eyelid (see **Fig. 2**), have been reported and are described in this text.[3,7]

Disfigurement, pain, bleeding, and drainage contribute to the morbidity of cutaneous metastases. Shimozuma and colleagues[8] found that cutaneous metastases had the greatest impact on quality of life in women with advanced or recurrent breast

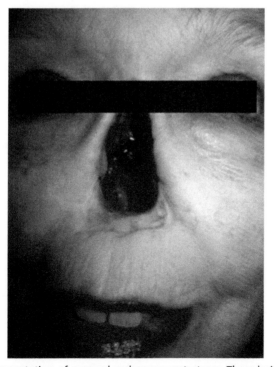

Fig. 4. Unusual presentation of mucosal melanoma metastases. These lesions are in-transit metastases from the original tumor, which presented in the nasal mucosa.

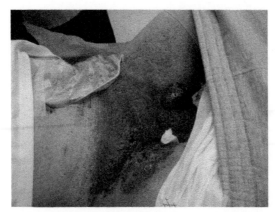

Fig. 5. Extensive cutaneous metastases from perianal mucosal melanoma.

cancer. Because skin involvement typically implies widespread disease, palliation is frequently the goal of therapy. With that being said, newer cancer immunotherapies have exhibited efficacy.

MELANOMA

Malignant melanoma is the most common cancer to metastasize to the skin (see **Figs. 1–6**).[3,9] The typical clinical appearance is a pigmented papule or nodule (see **Fig. 1**),

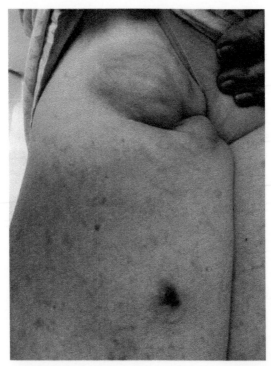

Fig. 6. Melanoma with bulky nodal disease and dermal intralymphatic metastases. The primary melanoma was located on the right calf.

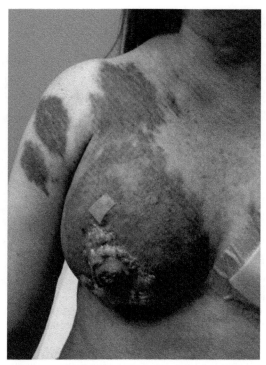

Fig. 7. Classic presentation of "inflammatory breast cancer," including rapid onset of erythema, edema, and peau d'orange appearance of the skin covering more than one-third of the breast.

although amelanotic lesions have been also reported.[10] These lesions can often progress in size, ulcerate, and bleed leading to significant patient morbidity.[10]

The incidence of skin metastasis in patients with melanoma ranges from 2% to 20%[11–13]; however, a more recent study of 2865 patients reported an incidence of 18%.[10] In comparison, sentinel lymph node positivity ranges from 14% to 30%.[14,15]

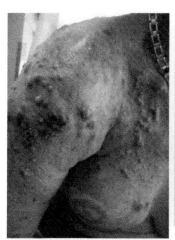
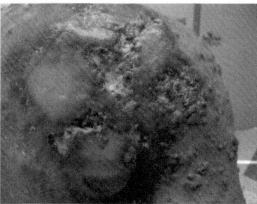

Fig. 8. Progressive carcinoma en cuirasse with ulcerated nodules.

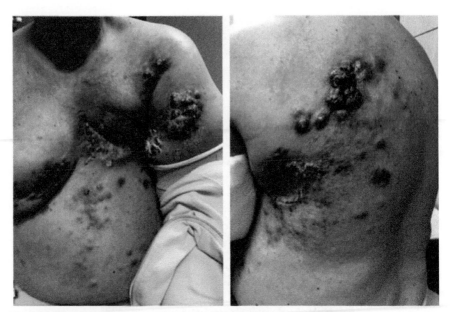

Fig. 9. Bulky breast cancer cutaneous metastases. Note extension along surgical and radiation borders. She also developed lesions along lymphedematous left arm.

Both skin and nodal disease have significant prognostic implications, thus they are important elements of melanoma staging.

Like all cancers, staging of melanoma uses the Tumor, Nodes, Metastasis (TNM) classification system per the American Joint Committee on Cancer (AJCC), which has made several changes in the eighth edition of the AJCC staging manual.[16] For the T category, the Breslow thickness of the primary tumor at intervals of 1, 2, and 4 mm to the nearest 0.1 mm (not 0.01 mm) and the presence or absence of ulceration are accounted for. Mitotic rate is no longer used for staging, although still reported and an important prognostic factor.

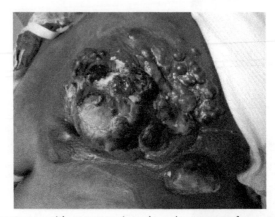

Fig. 10. Fungating tumor with numerous intradermal metastases from recurrent and metastatic breast cancer. This presentation is generally at the end of life.

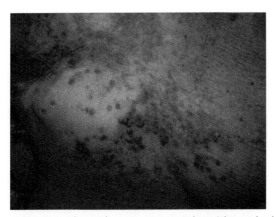

Fig. 11. Carcinoma telangiectoides with numerous pseudovesicles and telangiectasias.

The N category documents metastatic disease in both regional lymph nodes and non-nodal locoregional sites, including microsatellite, satellite, or in-transit metastases.[16] The definition of a microsatellite is disease that is microscopically discontinuous, either adjacent or deep, from the primary tumor. A satellite is metastatic disease occurring within 2 cm of the primary tumor. An in-transit metastasis is disease occurring more than 2 cm from the primary tumor, but not beyond the first echelon of region lymph nodes (see **Figs. 3** and **4**). Microsatellites, satellites, and in-transit metastases represent intralymphatic disease and outcomes are measured by nodal status, rather than the exact type of intralymphatic disease. These locoregional metastases are accounted for in the N category and herald stage III disease. In contrast, distant skin metastasis (beyond the first echelon of lymph nodes) is considered in the M category and heralds stage IV disease with a poor prognosis (see **Figs. 1**, **5**, and **6**).[17] Within the subgrouping of stage III patients (with intralymphatic disease), a significant amount of heterogeneity exists: 5-year survival ranges from 93% in patients with stage IIIA disease to 32% in patients with stage IIID disease (**Table 1**).[16]

The M category is assigned based on the anatomic site of metastasis (eg, skin vs lung). Additionally, it also accounts for serum lactate dehydrogenase (LDH) levels (elevated vs not elevated). For instance, a patient with a distant skin metastasis and low LDH would categorized as M1a(0). If the same patient had an elevated LDH, he or she would be classified as M1a(1).

Table 1
Differences in survival of metastatic melanoma within the stage III grouping

Stage	5 y, %	10 y, %
IIIA	93	88
IIIB	83	77
IIIC	69	60
IIID	32	24

Adapted from Gershenwald JE, Scolyer RA, Hess KR, et al. Melanoma staging: evidence-based changes in the American Joint Committee on Cancer eighth edition cancer staging manual. CA Cancer J Clin 2017;67(6):472–92; with permission.

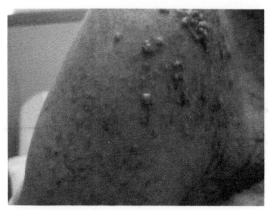

Fig. 12. Another example of carcinoma telangiectoides.

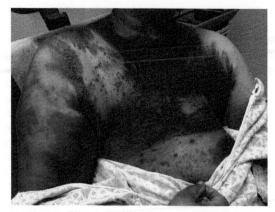

Fig. 13. Extensive cutaneous metastases with features of both carcinoma telangiectoides and carcinoma erysipeloides.

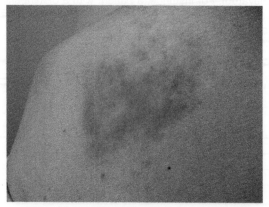

Fig. 14. Carcinoma erysipeloides. Breast cancer metastases with rashlike appearance. This patient was treated with several courses of antibiotics for cellulitis, delaying diagnosis of disease recurrence.

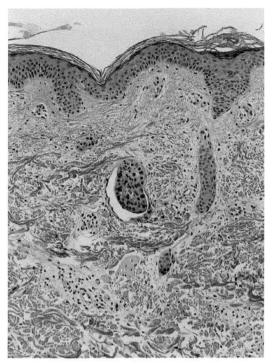

Fig. 15. Rashlike carcinoma erysipeloides presentation of dermal metastases demonstrates dilation of intravascular and intralymphatic vessels (hematoxylin-eosin, original magnification ×10).

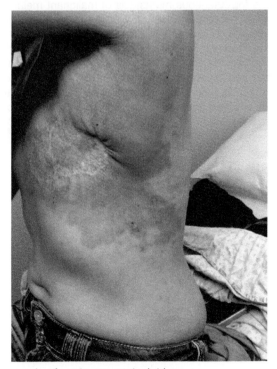

Fig. 16. Another example of carcinoma erysipeloides.

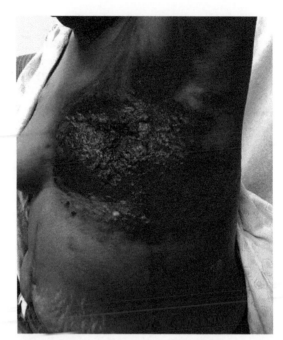

Fig. 17. Carcinoma en cuirasse with indurated scarlike plaques.

Treatment options for cutaneous metastasis of malignant melanoma has evolved over time from surgical resection and palliative radiation to systemic immunotherapies and/or targeted therapies. Talimogene laherparepvec (T-VEC), an oncolytic viral therapy approved by the Food and Drug Administration in 2015, is a modified herpes simplex virus that can be injected directly into the tumors and lymph nodes. The oncolytic activity of the virus is also believed to have the capacity of generating an abscopal, or bystander, effect in which distant tumors regress concomitantly with the treated tumor.[18] It is currently believed that the abscopal effect occurs due to a systemic anti-tumor immune response that is produced by adaptive immunity. T-VEC clinical trials

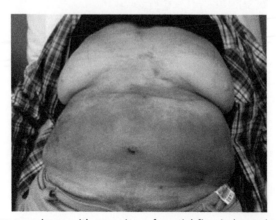

Fig. 18. Carcinoma en cuirasse with near circumferential firm indurated plaques.

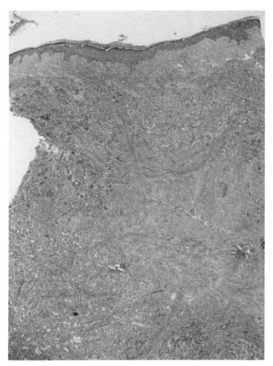

Fig. 19. Histology of carcinoma en cuirasse shows dense collagen stroma with infiltrating cords of tumor cells (hematoxylin-eosin, original magnification ×4).

demonstrated that when injected into cutaneous metastases, 34% of uninjected skin lesions and 15% of visceral lesions (also uninjected) demonstrated significant clinical response.[19] These results highlight the importance of the skin as an immune organ and its anti-tumor capability.

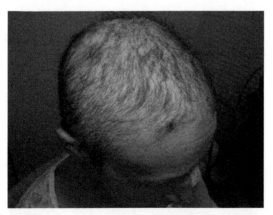

Fig. 20. Alopecia neoplastica from breast cancer showing patchy hair loss and few larger tumors. She had extensive infiltration of tumor cells in the scalp as well as liver, lung, and brain metastases. Of note, this patient used a cooling cap during her initial chemotherapy, which likely contributed to the scalp lesions but is unlikely to be responsible for the disease recurrence.

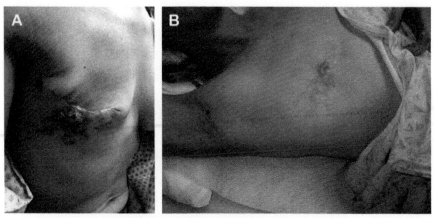

Fig. 21. (*A, B*) Breast cancer may recur within mastectomy scars.

BREAST CANCER

In women, breast cancer (see **Fig. 7**) is the most common primary cancer to metastasize to the skin (see **Figs. 2**, **3**, and 8–25).[2,3] Metastases typically appear on the anterior chest wall, typically from lymphatic extension to the overlying skin, in the form of skin-colored nodules (see **Figs. 8–10**).[20,21] Among the histologic subtypes of breast cancer, adenocarcinoma has the highest rate of skin metastasis, ranging from 77%

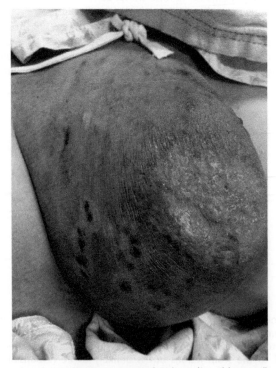

Fig. 22. Extensive cutaneous metastases presenting in radiated breast (breast cancer).

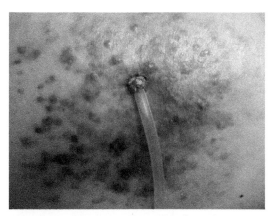

Fig. 23. Cutaneous metastases of breast cancer arising from direct extension through catheter tract (malignant pleural effusion).

to 82% of cases.[2,3] Perhaps owing to breast cancer's staggering overall prevalence and/or its propensity for skin involvement (see **Figs. 13–15**), it has been associated with a number of well-described clinical manifestations, including carcinoma erysipeloides, carcinoma telangiectoides, carcinoma en cuirasse, and alopecia neoplastica; each of which are described here in order of prevalence (provided in parenthesis).[22]

Carcinoma telangiectoides (11.2%) (see **Figs. 11–13**) occurs due to malignant spread via dermal lymphatics and presents as an erythematous patch with prominent telangiectasia and/or pseudovesicles on the chest that resembles lymphangioma circumscriptum.[23] Carcinoma telangiectoides may also appear on the face.[23] Carcinoma erysipeloides (3%) (see **Figs. 13–16**) is also due to lymphatic spread (see **Fig. 15**) and appears clinically as a fixed erythematous patch or plaque on the chest that resembles cellulitis or erysipelas.[23,24] Carcinoma en cuirasse (3%) (see **Figs. 17–19**) is characterized by thoracic wall lesions in the form of erythematous foci with induration, similar to scleroderma.[25] This unique name refers to the sclerotic nature of the disease, which refers to the cuirass, the metal breastplate worn by French cavalry in the nineteenth century. Alopecia neoplastica (2%) (see **Fig. 20**) is the loss of hair, resembling alopecia areata, due to invasion of malignant cells. Although carcinoma telangiectoides,

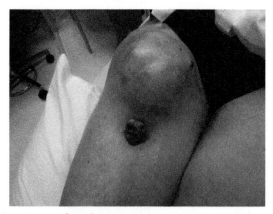

Fig. 24. Rare cystic metastasis from breast cancer.

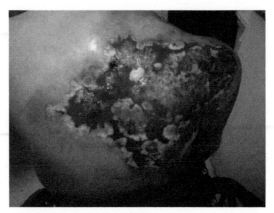

Fig. 25. Unusual presentations of erosive cutaneous metastatic breast cancer.

carcinoma erysipeloides, and alopecia neoplastica can be appreciated in other types of metastatic cancer (see **Fig. 32** depicts alopecia neoplastica in B-cell lymphoma), these conditions are most commonly associated with metastatic breast cancer.[22,26]

The implication of local skin involvement of a noninflammatory breast cancer is a T4b classification, thus automatic designation of stage III malignancy. In 2014, Silverman and colleagues[27] suggested that skin involvement should not override primary tumor size and lymph node involvement because it has caused a wide 5-year survival range in the stage III grouping. The T4b classification also requires ulceration of the skin or macroscopic nodules that are discontinuous with the primary tumor. These two requirements are new to the eighth edition of the AJCC Cancer Staging Manual and are meant to prevent inadvertent upstaging due to microscopic dermal satellites. An M1 classification in the M category is established in the presence of a distant metastasis, in the skin or otherwise, which ultimately merits stage IV disease.[28]

OTHER SOLID TUMORS

A review of literature by Kovacs and colleagues[29,30] reported that an overall incidence of cutaneous metastasis of 2.9% in cases of primary solid visceral malignancies. The

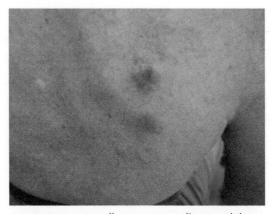

Fig. 26. Lung cancer metastases generally present as solitary nodules.

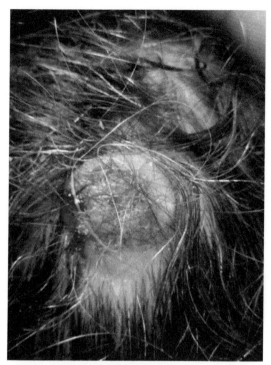

Fig. 27. Renal cell metastases on the scalp.

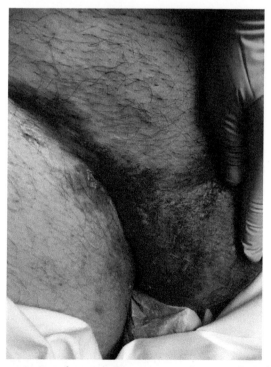

Fig. 28. Cutaneous metastases from colon cancer presenting as groin rash, initially treated as intertrigo.

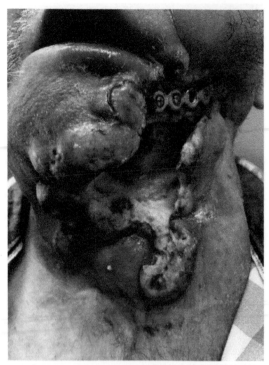

Fig. 29. Cancer extension into the skin with ulcerations in recurrent floor of mouth head and neck cancer.

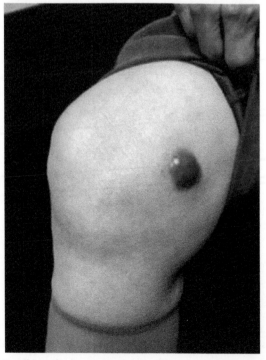

Fig. 30. Recurrent B-cell lymphoma presenting as solitary cutaneous metastases.

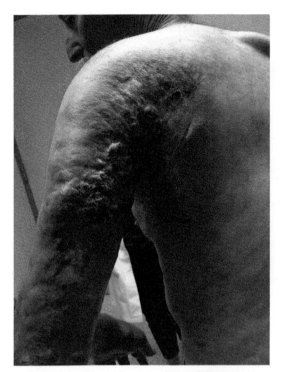

Fig. 31. Extensive cutaneous metastases from B-cell lymphoma.

investigators determined that lung, renal, and colorectal cancer have a metastatic preference for the skin, implying a biologic predilection for skin metastasis in these cancers. In contrast, this group reported a negative preference in gastric, liver, and pancreatic cancers.[31]

Lung

Lung cancer is the cause of 1.8% to 7.6% of cases of cutaneous metastasis and, in men, has been reported at a higher incidence than melanoma (see **Fig. 26**).[21,29] Current data suggest lung cancer is indeed the second most frequent cause of cutaneous metastasis

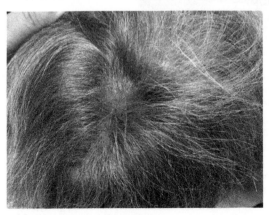

Fig. 32. Alopecia neoplastica from B-cell lymphoma.

Origin of cutaneous metastasis in women

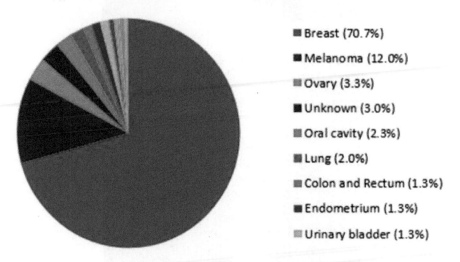

- Breast (70.7%)
- Melanoma (12.0%)
- Ovary (3.3%)
- Unknown (3.0%)
- Oral cavity (2.3%)
- Lung (2.0%)
- Colon and Rectum (1.3%)
- Endometrium (1.3%)
- Urinary bladder (1.3%)

Origin of cutaneous metastasis in men

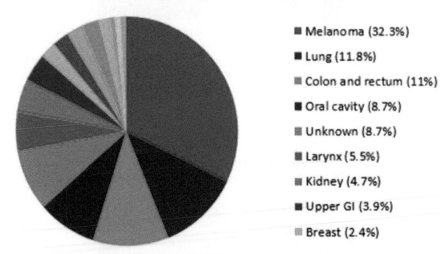

- Melanoma (32.3%)
- Lung (11.8%)
- Colon and rectum (11%)
- Oral cavity (8.7%)
- Unknown (8.7%)
- Larynx (5.5%)
- Kidney (4.7%)
- Upper GI (3.9%)
- Breast (2.4%)

Fig. 33. Origin of cutaneous metastasis stratified by sex. (*Data from* Lookingbill DP, Spangler N, Helm KF. Cutaneous metastases in patients with metastatic carcinoma: a retrospective study of 4020 patients. J Am Acad Dermatol 1993;29(2 Pt 1):228–36.)

in men, behind malignant melanoma. The malignant lesions tend to appear near the primary tumor, typically at a location on the thorax that is above the level of the diaphragm (see **Fig. 26**). Like most cutaneous metastases, there are frequently additional metastases to other organs at the time of diagnosis.[29,32] There are some data to suggest cancer of the upper lobes are the most likely to metastasize to the skin.[33,34] Large cell carcinoma and adenocarcinoma are the most common histologic types to produce skin metastases, whereas small cell carcinoma is a less frequent cause.[3,21,32,34]

Life expectancy at time of diagnosis stratified by cancer type

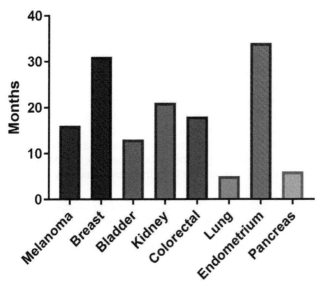

Fig. 34. Average life expectancy following diagnosis of cutaneous metastasis by cancer type. (*Data from* Lookingbill DP, Spangler N, Helm KF. Cutaneous metastases in patients with metastatic carcinoma: a retrospective study of 4020 patients. J Am Acad Dermatol 1993;29(2 Pt 1):228–36.)

Renal

Due to its indolent course, 1 in 3 cases of renal cell carcinoma (RCC) are at an advanced stage on initial presentation and, depending on the size of the primary tumor, between 4.8% and 18.4% of cases will have synchronous metastasis (metastasis at the time of presentation) (see **Fig. 27**).[35,36] Kidney cancer accounts for 4% to 8% of all cases of cutaneous metastases and 1.4% of cases of metastatic RCC will have skin involvement, with clear cell RCC being the most common histologic subtype found in metastatic RCC.[3,21,31,37,38] Although the trunk is the most common location of skin metastasis, interestingly, the scalp appears to be a preferred location for RCC (see **Fig. 27**).[37,39] RCC classically spreads hematogenously, and the path from the kidney to the scalp is made possible via inverted flow through the plexus of Batson to vertebral then emissary scalp veins.[39] Clinically, metastatic nodules frequently possess a black, brown, or purple color due to the highly vascular nature of RCC.[1]

Treatment of metastatic RCC is complicated by the fact that it is largely unresponsive to conventional chemotherapeutics, which also applies to metastatic disease of the skin.[38,40] The first-line combination therapy for metastatic RCC includes sunitinib, pazopanib, and bevacizumab with interferon-alpha.[38] With the exception of interferon-alpha, this regimen targets the vascular endothelial growth factor signaling axis.[38]

Colorectal Cancer Figure and Sister Mary Joseph Nodule

Another common cause of cutaneous metastasis is colorectal cancer (see **Fig. 26**). In 1993, Lookingbill and colleagues[3] reported that colorectal cancer accounted for 11% of all cutaneous metastases in men and 1.3% in women. Interestingly, the investigators noted that most of these patients had metastases located at abdominal incision sites (following colectomy). The most frequent sites of cutaneous metastasis appear to be the trunk, extremities, and perineum (see **Fig. 28**).[3] Cases of scalp and possible gingiva involvement have also been reported.[3,41]

Sister Mary Joseph Nodule is a rarely seen, but often cited, skin manifestation of metastatic disease. Sister Mary Joseph Dempsey, for whom this condition is named, was Dr William Mayo's surgical assistant who noted the association between paraumbilical nodules and metastatic intra-abdominal disease. With an estimated incidence of 1% to 3% of patients with an intra-abdominal and/or pelvic malignancy, this finding typically presents clinically as firm 0.5-cm to 2.0-cm umbilical nodule(s) in a female patient that can be painful or ulcerated. It may also drain pus, blood, or serous discharge.[42,43] The two most common cancer origins are gastrointestinal (52%) and gynecologic (28%) and among the gastrointestinal cancers, stomach (45%), colorectal (29%), and pancreatic (17%) cancers are the most frequently implicated.[43]

Head and Neck Cancer

Distant skin metastases occur in 1% to 2% of patients with squamous cell carcinoma of the head and neck with skin metastases accounting for 10% to 15% of all distant metastatic lesions (see **Fig. 29**).[44] Kmucha and Troxel[45] outline 3 possible mechanisms of metastatic spread of these tumors, which can be applied to most all cancer metastases: direct spread (through fascial planes), local spread (through dermal lymphatics), and distant spread (hematogenous spread). The most common mechanism of skin involvement in head and neck cancer is direct tumor extension into skin (see **Fig. 29**). However, many investigators do not consider direct extension to be a true metastasis.[44,45] Additionally, implantation of tumor cells along excision margins has been reported, which also should not necessarily be classified as metastatic disease.[44] Correct classification of metastasis is important because noncontiguous spread carries a worse prognosis.[6] Breast cancer also frequently exhibits direct extension, and the prognostic implications are discussed in the breast cancer subsection of this text.

HEMATOLOGIC MALIGNANCY

Leukemia cutis refers to extramedullary infiltration of neoplastic leukocytes into skin, resulting in clinically identifiable cutaneous lesions (see **Figs. 20–32**). In contrast to primary cutaneous lymphomas (eg, mycosis fungoides, a cutaneous T-cell lymphoma), the malignant cells in leukemia cutis do not normally have a predilection for the skin. Acute myeloid leukemia (AML) is the most likely hematologic malignancy to infiltrate the skin, with a prevalence of 2% to 4% in patients with AML.[46,47] Although cases associated with AML are more frequently reported, chronic lymphocytic leukemia (CLL) is a far more prevalent disease and produces leukemia cutis at similar rates; thus, CLL is likely more frequent overall cause.[47] Additionally, adult T-cell leukemia/lymphoma is also frequently implicated.[48]

Metastatic lesions in leukemia cutis have no clear anatomic preference and are clinically nonspecific, commonly appearing as papules, nodules, plaques, or tumors with wide variations in color (see **Figs. 20** and **31**).[47] Diagnosis can be complicated in leukemic patients because of more frequent skin changes that are related to altered hematopoiesis (eg, purpura due to thrombocytopenia) and/or paraneoplastic disorders (eg, Sweet syndrome). Further complicating diagnosis, neoplastic cells have been found in skin changes that are unrelated to the patient's malignancy, such as squamous cell skin cancer, psoriasis, and herpes simplex infection.[49–51] Presence of these neoplastic cells should not be considered leukemia cutis. Histopathologic diagnosis along with hematologic studies (eg, peripheral smear) and clinical course are essential to make a conclusive diagnosis of leukemia cutis.[47]

GENERAL APPROACH TO THERAPY

A review article by Wong and colleagues[20] in 2013 recommended excision of cutaneous metastases when surgically feasible and when it will result in a significant decrease in total tumor burden, improve the quality of life, or increase functionality. Using metastatic melanoma as a model, the investigators suggested 1-cm excision margins, with the caveat that no great data exists regarding excision margins of metastatic disease.[20]

In general, treatment follows the regimen appropriate for the primary metastatic malignancy. However, systemic therapy appears to have limited efficacy.[52,53] Therefore, skin-directed therapies have been developed to treat skin metastases. Skin-directed therapies are forms of localized treatment that have been shown to illicit a greater response than systemic therapy alone.[53] A meta-analysis by Spratt and colleagues[53] reported high response rates and low recurrence rates following skin-directed therapy. The modalities of skin-directed therapies include electrochemotherapy, photodynamic therapy, radiotherapy, intralesional therapy, and topical therapy, of which electrochemotherapy appears to be the most efficacious.[53] Electrochemotherapy functions via the application of pulsed electricity to a tumor-specific area to increase cell permeability. It has been shown to significantly increase the cytotoxicity of cisplatin and bleomycin.[20] Another efficacious skin-directed therapy is radiotherapy, which is a highly accurate modality that has also long been associated with the abscopal effect.[54]

SUMMARY

It is understood that cutaneous metastases tend to appear on the skin overlying the region of the primary tumor, a phenomenon that has been best described in lung and breast cancer.[3] However, these regional skin metastases are certainly not always the case. In the case of RCC, its aggressive propensity to spread hematogenously allows neoplastic cells to appear on the scalp (see **Fig. 27**).[39] Although breast cancer may also appear on the scalp, in a clinical condition termed *alopecia neoplastica* (see **Fig. 20**), it prefers to travel via lymphatics to local skin. This behavior has led to a number of clinical descriptions that are virtually pathognomonic for cutaneous metastases of breast cancer, such as *carcinoma en cuirasse* (see **Figs. 17–19**). Among all invasive cancers, science has been able to extract a wealth of information from metastatic melanoma. Its lymphatic spread can be readily visualized in the form of an in-transit metastasis (see **Fig. 3**), photoacoustic tomography can detect metastatic cells traveling in the circulation, and its high mutational burden renders it susceptible to innovative immunotherapies.[55,56]

Malignant cells often use pathways intended for immune-cell trafficking to grant themselves access to lymphatics, vasculature, and ultimately non-native tissues.[57] To do so, they must undergo a number of cellular changes to gain trafficking capabilities, many of which are already readily available in immune cells. Immunotherapy aims to exploit the immune system's ability to traffic into any tissue and eliminate unfriendly cells with remarkable specificity. Exhaustive study in this field has been spent discovering methods to encourage the immune system to target tumor cells and subsequently activate a systemic antitumor immune response. Finding such a method has proven to be an uphill battle, partially because cancer cells often possess immune-evasion mechanisms, such as programmed cell death ligand 1 (PD-1). Given the skin's high density of adaptive immune cells, it comes as no surprise that recent advances in immunotherapy (eg, PD-1 inhibitors and T-VEC) have demonstrated efficacy in the treatment of cutaneous metastases.[58,59]

REFERENCES

1. Alcaraz I, Cerroni L, Rutten A, et al. Cutaneous metastases from internal malignancies: a clinicopathologic and immunohistochemical review. Am J Dermatopathol 2012;34(4):347–93.
2. Gan EY, Chio MT, Tan WP. A retrospective review of cutaneous metastases at the National Skin Centre Singapore. Australas J Dermatol 2015;56(1):1–6.
3. Lookingbill DP, Spangler N, Helm KF. Cutaneous metastases in patients with metastatic carcinoma: a retrospective study of 4020 patients. J Am Acad Dermatol 1993;29(2 Pt 1):228–36.
4. Nashan D, Meiss F, Braun-Falco M, et al. Cutaneous metastases from internal malignancies. Dermatol Ther 2010;23(6):567–80.
5. Saeed S, Keehn CA, Morgan MB. Cutaneous metastasis: a clinical, pathological, and immunohistochemical appraisal. J Cutan Pathol 2004;31(6):419–30.
6. Cole RD, McGuirt WF. Prognostic significance of skin involvement from mucosal tumors of the head and neck. Arch Otolaryngol Head Neck Surg 1995;121(11):1246–8.
7. Bianciotto C, Demirci H, Shields CL, et al. Metastatic tumors to the eyelid: report of 20 cases and review of the literature. Arch Ophthalmol 2009;127(8):999–1005.
8. Shimozuma K, Sonoo H, Ichihara K. Analysis of the factors influencing the quality of life of patients with advanced or recurrent breast cancer. Surg Today 1995;25(10):874–82.
9. Wong CY, Helm MA, Helm TN, et al. Patterns of skin metastases: a review of 25 years' experience at a single cancer center. Int J Dermatol 2014;53(1):56–60.
10. Savoia P, Fava P, Nardo T, et al. Skin metastases of malignant melanoma: a clinical and prognostic survey. Melanoma Res 2009;19(5):321–6.
11. Aitken DR, James AG, Carey LC. Local cutaneous recurrence after conservative excision of malignant melanoma. Arch Surg 1984;119(6):643–6.
12. Cascinelli N, Bufalino R, Marolda R, et al. Regional non-nodal metastases of cutaneous melanoma. Eur J Surg Oncol 1986;12(2):175–80.
13. Heenan PJ, Ghaznawie M. The pathogenesis of local recurrence of melanoma at the primary excision site. Br J Plast Surg 1999;52(3):209–13.
14. Morton DL, Thompson JF, Cochran AJ, et al. Final trial report of sentinel-node biopsy versus nodal observation in melanoma. N Engl J Med 2014;370(7):599–609.
15. van der Ploeg AP, van Akkooi AC, Rutkowski P, et al. Prognosis in patients with sentinel node-positive melanoma is accurately defined by the combined Rotterdam tumor load and Dewar topography criteria. J Clin Oncol 2011;29(16):2206–14.
16. Gershenwald JE, Scolyer RA, Hess KR, et al. Melanoma staging: evidence-based changes in the American Joint Committee on Cancer eighth edition cancer staging manual. CA Cancer J Clin 2017;67(6):472–92.
17. Pan Y, Haydon AM, McLean CA, et al. Prognosis associated with cutaneous melanoma metastases. Australas J Dermatol 2015;56(1):25–8.

18. Mole RH. Whole body irradiation; radiobiology or medicine? Br J Radiol 1953; 26(305):234–41.
19. Andtbacka RH, Kaufman HL, Collichio F, et al. Talimogene laherparepvec improves durable response rate in patients with advanced melanoma. J Clin Oncol 2015;33(25):2780–8.
20. Wong CY, Helm MA, Kalb RE, et al. The presentation, pathology, and current management strategies of cutaneous metastasis. N Am J Med Sci 2013;5(9): 499–504.
21. Brownstein MH, Helwig EB. Patterns of cutaneous metastasis. Arch Dermatol 1972;105(6):862–8.
22. Patra S, Khandpur S, Khanna N, et al. Angioma like carcinoma telangiectoides: an unusual presentation of breast carcinoma metastasis. Indian J Dermatol Venereol Leprol 2018;84(1):83–5.
23. Marneros AG, Blanco F, Husain S, et al. Classification of cutaneous intravascular breast cancer metastases based on immunolabeling for blood and lymph vessels. J Am Acad Dermatol 2009;60(4):633–8.
24. Al Ameer A, Imran M, Kaliyadan F, et al. Carcinoma erysipeloides as a presenting feature of breast carcinoma: a case report and brief review of literature. Indian Dermatol Online J 2015;6(6):396–8.
25. Arapovic SJ, Simic L. Cutaneous metastases—carcinoma en cuirasse. Acta Dermatovenerol Croat 2002;10(3):167–70.
26. Conner KB, Cohen PR. Cutaneous metastasis of breast carcinoma presenting as alopecia neoplastica. South Med J 2009;102(4):385–9.
27. Silverman D, Ruth K, Sigurdson ER, et al. Skin involvement and breast cancer: are T4b lesions of all sizes created equal? J Am Coll Surg 2014;219(3): 534–44.
28. Giuliano AE, Edge SB, Hortobagyi GN. Eighth edition of the AJCC cancer staging manual: breast cancer. Ann Surg Oncol 2018;25(7):1783–5.
29. Kovacs KA, Hegedus B, Kenessey I, et al. Tumor type-specific and skin region-selective metastasis of human cancers: another example of the "seed and soil" hypothesis. Cancer Metastasis Rev 2013;32(3–4):493–9.
30. Mueller TJ, Wu H, Greenberg RE, et al. Cutaneous metastases from genitourinary malignancies. Urology 2004;63(6):1021–6.
31. Kovacs KA, Kenessey I, Timar J. Skin metastasis of internal cancers: a single institution experience. Pathol Oncol Res 2013;19(3):515–20.
32. Hidaka T, Ishii Y, Kitamura S. Clinical features of skin metastasis from lung cancer. Intern Med 1996;35(6):459–62.
33. Coslett LM, Katlic MR. Lung cancer with skin metastasis. Chest 1990;97(3): 757–9.
34. Pajaziti L, Hapciu SR, Dobruna S, et al. Skin metastases from lung cancer: a case report. BMC Res Notes 2015;8:139.
35. Lughezzani G, Jeldres C, Isbarn H, et al. Tumor size is a determinant of the rate of stage T1 renal cell cancer synchronous metastasis. J Urol 2009;182(4):1287–93.
36. Graves A, Hessamodini H, Wong G, et al. Metastatic renal cell carcinoma: update on epidemiology, genetics, and therapeutic modalities. Immunotargets Ther 2013;2:73–90.
37. Held B, Johnson DE. Cutaneous metastases from malignant genitourinary disease. South Med J 1972;65(5):569–71.
38. Hsieh JJ, Purdue MP, Signoretti S, et al. Renal cell carcinoma. Nat Rev Dis Primers 2017;3:17009.

39. Errami M, Margulis V, Huerta S. Renal cell carcinoma metastatic to the scalp. Rare Tumors 2016;8(4):6400.

40. Pantuck AJ, Zisman A, Belldegrun AS. The changing natural history of renal cell carcinoma. J Urol 2001;166(5):1611–23.

41. Wang DY, Ye F, Lin JJ, et al. Cutaneous metastasis: a rare phenomenon of colorectal cancer. Ann Surg Treat Res 2017;93(5):277–80.

42. Piura B, Meirovitz M, Bayme M, et al. Sister Mary Joseph's nodule originating from endometrial carcinoma incidentally detected during surgery for an umbilical hernia: a case report. Arch Gynecol Obstet 2006;274(6):385–8.

43. Galvan VG. Sister Mary Joseph's nodule. Ann Intern Med 1998;128(5):410.

44. Pitman KT, Johnson JT. Skin metastases from head and neck squamous cell carcinoma: incidence and impact. Head Neck 1999;21(6):560–5.

45. Kmucha ST, Troxel JM. Dermal metastases in epidermoid carcinoma of the head and neck. Arch Otolaryngol Head Neck Surg 1993;119(3):326–30.

46. Agis H, Weltermann A, Fonatsch C, et al. A comparative study on demographic, hematological, and cytogenetic findings and prognosis in acute myeloid leukemia with and without leukemia cutis. Ann Hematol 2002;81(2):90–5.

47. Wagner G, Fenchel K, Back W, et al. Leukemia cutis—epidemiology, clinical presentation, and differential diagnoses. J Dtsch Dermatol Ges 2012;10(1):27–36.

48. Tokura Y, Sawada Y, Shimauchi T. Skin manifestations of adult T-cell leukemia/lymphoma: clinical, cytological and immunological features. J Dermatol 2014;41(1): 19–25.

49. Dargent JL, Kornreich A, Andre L, et al. Cutaneous infiltrate of chronic lymphocytic leukemia surrounding a primary squamous cell carcinoma of the skin. Report of an additional case and reflection on its pathogenesis. J Cutan Pathol 1998;25(9):479–80.

50. Metzler G, Cerroni L, Schmidt H, et al. Leukemic cells within skin lesions of psoriasis in a patient with acute myelogenous leukemia. J Cutan Pathol 1997;24(7): 445–8.

51. Ziemer M, Bornkessel A, Hahnfeld S, et al. 'Specific' cutaneous infiltrate of B-cell chronic lymphocytic leukemia at the site of a florid herpes simplex infection. J Cutan Pathol 2005;32(8):581–4.

52. Richtig E, Ludwig R, Kerl H, et al. Organ- and treatment-specific local response rates to systemic and local treatment modalities in stage IV melanoma. Br J Dermatol 2005;153(5):925–31.

53. Spratt DE, Gordon Spratt EA, Wu S, et al. Efficacy of skin-directed therapy for cutaneous metastases from advanced cancer: a meta-analysis. J Clin Oncol 2014;32(28):3144–55.

54. Cotter SE, Dunn GP, Collins KM, et al. Abscopal effect in a patient with metastatic Merkel cell carcinoma following radiation therapy: potential role of induced antitumor immunity. Arch Dermatol 2011;147(7):870–2.

55. Xia J, Yao J, Wang LV. Photoacoustic tomography: principles and advances. Electromagn Waves (Camb) 2014;147:1–22.

56. Furney SJ, Turajlic S, Stamp G, et al. The mutational burden of acral melanoma revealed by whole-genome sequencing and comparative analysis. Pigment Cell Melanoma Res 2014;27(5):835–8.

57. Koizumi K, Hojo S, Akashi T, et al. Chemokine receptors in cancer metastasis and cancer cell-derived chemokines in host immune response. Cancer Sci 2007; 98(11):1652–8.

58. Blackmon JT, Stratton MS, Kwak Y, et al. Inflammatory melanoma in transit metastases with complete response to talimogene laherparepvec. JAAD Case Rep 2017;3(4):280–3.
59. Gulati N, Carvajal RD, Postow MA, et al. Definite regression of cutaneous melanoma metastases upon addition of topical contact sensitizer diphencyprone to immune checkpoint inhibitor treatment. Exp Dermatol 2016;25(7):553–4.

Moving?

Make sure your subscription moves with you!

To notify us of your new address, find your **Clinics Account Number** (located on your mailing label above your name), and contact customer service at:

Email: journalscustomerservice-usa@elsevier.com

800-654-2452 (subscribers in the U.S. & Canada)
314-447-8871 (subscribers outside of the U.S. & Canada)

Fax number: 314-447-8029

Elsevier Health Sciences Division
Subscription Customer Service
3251 Riverport Lane
Maryland Heights, MO 63043

*To ensure uninterrupted delivery of your subscription, please notify us at least 4 weeks in advance of move.

Printed and bound by CPI Group (UK) Ltd, Croydon, CR0 4YY

14/10/2024

01774062-0001